Menopause and Me

handling the emotional side

Barbara Frodsham

Menopause and Me
handling the emotional side

First published in 2010 by

Ecademy Press

48 St Vincent Drive, St Albans, Hertfordshire, AL1 5SJ

info@ecademy-press.com

www.ecademy-press.com

Printed and Bound by Lightning Source in the UK and USA

Set in Warnock Pro by Charlotte Mouncey

Printed on acid-free paper from managed forests.
This book is printed on demand, so no copies will be
remaindered or pulped.

ISBN 978-1-905823-75-8

A huge message of gratitude and appreciation to everyone who supported, helped and encouraged me to write this book.

Thank you.

I dedicate this book to every single menopausal woman who is fed up with being too hot!

You are not alone

And you will be fine!

Contents

Chapter 1

Purpose

I am writing this book to help women handle the emotional side of the menopause. There are many excellent books available, written from a physical perspective and medical perspective. I intend this to be a self-help book that you can dip into to help you to *handle how you feel* about the menopause, both in the moment and also to set yourself up for success in the long term.

It can be hard to deal with everyday life and carry on as usual with these unwelcome symptoms; sometimes they are in the background and at other times they are overwhelmingly front and centre. They can be constant reminders of age and, at times, make me feel very vulnerable and no longer as in control as I was once – quite the opposite to those teenage years when I knew everything, I was invincible and I had my whole life in front of me. There can be a temptation to just give in and let go, allowing ourselves to be at the mercy of our hormones. On the other hand, life has so much to offer now to women of a 'certain age'. I love that expression, it comes from the French and it is such an elegant way to talk about middle age. I fully intend to be in charge of my menopause, and to keep myself fit and healthy for as long as possible. I believe that taking charge of the menopause is all about attitude, and it is all about handling the emotional side of the menopause, as well as the physical aspects.

My goal is to help women to see their situation differently, discover new ways of coping and alternative ways of thinking to minimise the negative effects of this important and significant transition time of life. It would be easy to give in and let the symptoms get the better of us, but my aim is to help women to step into their power and take charge of their lives and themselves.

I believe that women who are going through the menopause right now are at the forefront of a new wave of women who are strong and capable, and who are just not willing to let their evolving biology get in their way. We really are making it up as we go along. Role models are few and far between. Our approach is a long way from those of the generation before who looked as if they bought a pleated skirt with an elasticated waist and a cardigan and then faded into the background.

Why me? My areas of expertise are in personal development, specifically teaching people how to think differently about their situation. Over the last 25 years, I've learned many tools and techniques for dealing with situations. One of my key skills is a deep understanding of how our thinking can sabotage us. I'm really good at working out what gets in the way for people and helping them to find ways to get over that. In any situation, attitude is key to making the most of it and getting the best from it.

I'll be drawing on my 25 years of experience in the world of learning and development and my knowledge of people and their behaviour, using ideas and concepts from many areas of study, including Neuro Linguistic Programming (NLP). Put simply, NLP is about the way we think, the language we use to describe our experiences and our world. It also looks at the programmes we run in our mind. We have lots of these programmes; for example, you'll probably have one for brushing your teeth: do you start in the middle or at the back, top or bottom first? It's likely that you brush your teeth the same way every day without even thinking about it. That's a programme: an automatic set of behaviours that achieve a desired result, every time. Generally these programmes work brilliantly for us; every now and then we can come across some that are not so effective. We can use NLP to create more useful or helpful programmes.

I am also in the middle of my menopausal change, feeling the symptoms on a daily basis and recognising how this change affects people in real time (as opposed to looking back at it after the fact, when it is easy to forget the smaller details)

The day I realised that I was menopausal was a terrific shock for me. I was completely unprepared for it. I didn't expect it and, if truth be told, I had sort of thought it wouldn't ever happen to me, not for at least another 10 years (I was 48). I'd mistakenly believed that I would be one of the women who would get it late and that it would all be over in no time.

I can remember on several occasions sitting next to particular friends (three of them and one of me) who were discussing the symptoms of the menopause and feeling completely detached from it. I saw them almost as if they were a different species from me! I would hear them talking about it and, although I was at the same table, I was a million miles away from them. They would take off layers of clothing and, soon afterwards, put them back on again, complain about being tired from lack of sleep and talk about the merits of herbs. I would drift away from their conversation as though it had absolutely nothing to do with me.

Looking back, I marvel at the fact that I could think that way and I'm rather surprised that it is a topic that is not really talked about in society – almost as if it were a taboo subject. Apparently, many mothers don't even talk to their daughters about it! I'm also rather ashamed that I didn't listen or try to understand their point of view. It really was a waste of their knowledge and experience. Now I'm hungry for every shred of information I can get!

Once I got over the initial shock, there came the realisation that it was probably too late for me to have children. I love children and always thought I would make a pretty good mother. But for years, in fact since I was about 18, I'd been saying, "Not now, but maybe in 10 years' time". The decades had gone by and now my fertile years were over; and even though I still did not want children at that point, it was an unwelcome fact that I no longer had a choice in the matter.

It took a while for the message to sink in but, as you know, there is nothing you can do to prevent it. The inevitable arrives and you have to deal with it. This book is about how to do that: helping you to handle that transition period and giving you tools, techniques and strategies to make it easier.

I've been talking to people, reading blogs and internet forums from women who are menopausal and many of them say, "I just want my Old Self back". What we know is this: our Old Self is not coming back. We can long for it and yearn for it, but that self is gone, we can only mourn it. However … we are about to become a new Old Self! A new Me is emerging.

This book is about offering you activities, exercises and ideas to help to shift your thinking, to take control and make the most of this new version of yourself.

What I am certainly beginning to come to terms with is that my old self will not be back. The change is upon me, it's a feature of the landscape. I have to move on and deal with life as it is, not as I would wish it to be. What I also know is that I can handle this better and perhaps do some things differently – and you can, too. I have a sense that handling emotions and feelings is the key to getting through this.

Note:

You may find some of the activities rather unusual. My initial thought was to suggest that you just complete those you like the look of, and perhaps try some of the others. However the more unusual activities may not be the type of thing that you normally tackle. Yet they might offer ways of thinking that are new and unfamiliar to you. So, in the spirit of thinking differently and getting new ideas: if you find there is an activity you are resisting, no matter why, then all the more reason for you to do it.

Some people comment on the activities I propose, saying, "I don't really do this sort of thing" or "I can't see myself doing this". I suggest that you just try one or two of these exercises to see what you get from them. Just give it a go and experiment. After all, you've got nothing to lose and perhaps many new insights to gain.

Do as much or as little as you feel like, but remember, you will get out of this what you put in. You alone can make the time you spend with this book the most useful, productive and life-changing time of your life.

When you set out to read this book there are a number of ways you can do it:

- You can read it from cover to cover, doing the activities as you go along

- You can dip into it, just open it at a page and see what relevance that topic has for you

- You could just do the activities alone

- You can decide which chapters you want to delve into and find out about

- Or you could read it all and then do the activities afterwards

The choice is yours, but whichever approach you take, it will definitely help you to take a new look at how you think and feel about yourself and the menopause.

Chapter 2

Start here

"You can't change what you don't acknowledge"

Dr Phil McGraw

America's Dr Phil says, "You can't change what you don't acknowledge". What I am suggesting here is that you completely acknowledge where you are in your life and that this perimenopause or menopause is actually happening, there is no denying it. The question is: Can you accept the challenge?

By the way, technically the menopause is when you have had one year without a period; before that, the change is called 'perimenopause'.

The menopause sneaks up on some people, seems to pass by unnoticed for a lucky few and, for others, it comes with the ferocity of a freak storm, but seems to last quite a bit longer. The very fact that you are reading this suggests that either you know it is on the horizon and you are learning and preparing for it, or the symptoms are more noticeable and you are looking for new ideas and ways to handle it. At the same time, there may be a tendency to look the other way and pretend it is not there, 'ignore it and it will go away'.

If I were being harsh, I'd say to you, "Get real. Stop pretending this menopause thing isn't happening, get clear on what the reality is for you. How is your life different now? How are you acting, feeling, behaving, seeing things, what are you saying to yourself?" But those questions are for much later in our quest. Just now, I'd like you to consider your own situation. Notice that there is the reality from your perspective, the way you see things and the way you see the world. Then there is also your environment: where you live, what surrounds you at home and perhaps at work. In the media we see powerful advertisements about looking good, looking after ourselves, make-up and diet. Nearly all the women in these ads look in their twenties. I'm told that adverts for weight-loss diets may feature models who have not yet reached their twenties. So often we are influenced to strive for something that is really outside of our reach. Recently, a Sunday newspaper supplement had a front cover that proclaimed 'Look younger: how to look your best without surgery!' I wonder if this implies that you can't look good if you don't look young. Have a think about the messages that our culture gives us about age, about the menopause and about women who are menopausal.

What are the messages that you receive from your environment, from your work, from your family and friends?

Some ideas of things to look out for are:

- Are the people around you sympathetic?

- Do they tease you?

- Do they support you?

- Do people assume you have gone a bit batty and not take you seriously?

Stuck in the Problem?

Sometimes people get stuck in the problem; they keep focusing on it and talking about it, without thinking about what they could do to make it better or looking for any solutions. When they think about it, or they talk to other people about it, they play a sort of 'tape recording', repeating the same things over and over again. I call this 'getting stuck in the story'. So, when someone tells and retells their story about the problem, and they only focus on only those few negative aspects of it, unwittingly, they reinforce the message by repeating it over and over again until they are unable to see any other way of looking at the situation.

For example: Samantha is in a relationship with someone she does not trust, he has had an affair with one of her close friends. She is constantly worried that he will do it again; if he is ever late home, she imagines he has gone off with someone else. She is miserable and has lost her sparkle. From an onlooker's perspective, it would be better if she cut her losses and left so that she could meet someone else and have a more fulfilling relationship. Whenever she talks about it though, she says she is scared to be on her own, she's not attractive enough, she'd never meet anyone else and, besides, how could she manage the mortgage? She's never been on her own before. This is the story that she tells over and over again; she believes it is true.

When someone does this, they are stuck in a rut. With this frame of mind, they can also find it difficult to listen to helpful suggestions from others, even though they are not happy with the situation. Some people even resist help altogether. I've been in a couple of situations where someone has wanted to help me to feel better, and they have made what could have been helpful suggestions, but I was in the mindset that says, 'You just don't understand how I feel, how can you come up with a solution when you just don't know what this is like?' and then I would dig in my heels and would not want to listen. Even though I was really unhappy, it's almost as if I didn't want someone else to solve the problem for me. In fact, I'd go even further and say that it seemed preferable to be stuck in the problem rather than to step into the scary unknown of the solution.

Are you using this as an excuse?

This is linked with the last point. Let's say we accept the status quo, the situation we are in, i.e. 'I am menopausal.' Then we look for the symptoms, which can be pretty easy to find and we could find plenty more if we tried. (There's a big list of them on page 212.) Then we could say, "Well, it's not my fault, this is the situation I am in and there is nothing I can do about it".

If this might be you, notice what your story is, what do you tell yourself? What do you say to other people about it? Do you find yourself saying the same things over and over again and not doing anything about it?

Liz complains frequently of not sleeping and being tired all the time. She has a demanding job and works really hard, her family is going through some problems that she is helping them with. She gets exhausted and has very little time for herself.

I suspect that her sleep problems are not only to do with the menopause but also to do with the fact that she is very stressed and does not relax much. However, in her mind it's all because of the menopause. Maybe it is and maybe it isn't, but when you use it as an excuse, you will easily find the evidence you need to prove yourself right.

What are you blindly accepting?

I read recently that a great many women wait for more than a year before going to get help when they realise they are menopausal. Maybe some of your symptoms have a remedy; maybe there is other type of help that is available to you. This book will give you ideas and thoughts about what you can do differently and what more you can do to help yourself.

It's OK, you will be fine

And you know, you really will be fine. You will be able to handle this the way you have already handled difficult times in your life. You've got this far and been able to cope with everything life has thrown at you. You might not know yet how you will deal with it but, as your best friend will probably tell you, "Don't worry, you will be fine!"

Attitude

"Attitude is a little thing that makes a big difference"
Winston Churchill

We know that the menopausal changes are going to happen, regardless of what we want, and often when we resist things it just makes it harder. You might as well be prepared and get ahead of the game! Here's an example:

Think about this: imagine you have a chore to do, let's use washing the car as an example.

When we resist it, it makes the job seem harder, we focus on how difficult and unpleasant it will be and we magnify all the negatives of the situation. We can easily imagine that a 20-minute job will take an hour and will be horrible. Also when we think like this we can often forget the original motivation we had to get the job done. For me, washing the car used to be a task of gargantuan proportions. In my mind, before I started I would imagine that I would get soaked, I would be cold and wet, I would break a nail, at least one if not more (and that's a drama in itself!) Somehow, the car in my mind appeared twice the size of the car in reality. I would picture bits of dirt that would be really stubborn to get off. Not to mention the wheels, hah! They would take ages and would never be quite clean enough. Plenty of negative feelings and thoughts about a task that I hadn't even begun!

Now imagine the same chore; this time you have decided you are going to enjoy it and find pleasure in it. You picture the job done well: the gleaming paintwork, the pristine bumpers, the shining wheels and the sparkling clean windscreen and windows. You take the job a step at a time. Roof first: brilliant, and congratulate yourself on doing a really good job with that, then you do the windows and smile to yourself as you see them glinting through the soapy water. Each panel, bumper and wheel gives you an opportunity to be pleased with yourself until the job is done.

You've probably washed a car or done similar such chores many times before, so you can draw on your own experience. When it comes to the menopause, this is a first time for you. You may not have thought about it this way before, so you might need to give yourself some time to think about what the good and positive things might be. In order to do that, you might need to be selfish about your own needs for a change, rather than always doing things for others and neglecting yourself.

A note about the word 'selfish'; some of us have been brought up to think that this is a bad thing, a really negative trait. If that is what you think, then it is unlikely that you will want to be selfish on purpose. You could try out the word I use when I mean taking time for myself so that I can recharge my batteries. I call it being 'me-ish'. Think about it like this: you need to look after yourself first so that you can take better care of others. If you are stressed and frazzled, then you are in no position to help anyone else.

It's hard to ignore it

Probably, when you go through the change, you will have to get used to the idea of doing things differently, feeling different and also acting differently. What is about to develop and flower and burst into being is a new You. Let me clarify: what will emerge during the menopausal process is not an 'old, worn-out You' as some people might describe it; rather you will find and discover a whole, lovely, new You.

And what you are, no doubt, coming to recognise about the menopause is that:

- You cannot ignore it: it is present with you every day and every hot flush, or cold moment, is another reminder of it

- You cannot change it: the process has started and you can't change the fact that it is happening, and will continue to its natural conclusion

- You cannot fight it, because then you are fighting with yourself and that is not healthy or wise

- You can push it back with HRT, though that comes with an element of risk and, besides, it will reappear when you stop the taking the hormones

Arguably, you can pretend it is not happening to you. I've seen many women out and about, dressed as if they were 20 years younger than they are. To the observer's eye comes the familiar phrase 'mutton dressed as lamb'. Now, I'm all for people making the best of themselves and keeping themselves young and fit. But there is a moment when trying to look young by wearing youthful dress and having a young hairstyle and make-up only serves to highlight age even more. The 'mask' or disguise that is used to hide the person's age becomes counter-productive. The very thing the person is seeking to hide becomes even more obvious. You might say, "Well, what does it matter if I want to pretend that I'm 30 or so, when I am 50?" I would say that, if you do, first of all you are perhaps not showing yourself at your best. You probably don't want people to be looking at you thinking 'Gosh, she's far too old to be wearing that!' It's a bit like when people who are overweight wear smaller-size clothes, imagining that it will make them a smaller size – but the tighter clothes just make the person look bigger. However, if a woman is wearing clothing that is the correct size, carefully chosen, she can appear much slimmer. Next time you are out and about, take a look at the women who look great and seem happy in themselves. What do you notice and admire about them?

The other reason this matters is that you are not being who you really are, not being true to yourself and, at some level, you are lying to yourself and to others.

How do I look?

Then there is the tricky topic of surgery, Botox and other 'enhancements'. A photographer told me that when we look at someone's face who has had that type of treatment, we take in the work they have had done, make a calculation in our heads as if to say, 'They've had this amount of Botox/plastic surgery, therefore they are probably about x age'. We are, apparently, pretty good at this. For example, we look at a woman who is around 55 who has had plastic surgery, and let's say the lines on her face now make her look as if she is 45. We notice this, then we evaluate the totality of how the person looks, their skin tone/ texture, the fluidity of how they move and how they sound, then we recalibrate them back to the original age, saying things like 'She looks great for her age'. Curiously, when younger people have had plastic surgery, this recalibration can end up making them seem older than they really are.

All this assumes that you are actually bothered about what other people think; maybe you are not, which is fine, too. And besides, there is nothing wrong with wanting to look younger, or to look less lined; the question is: Who are you fooling?

For the whole time I have been writing this book, I have been trying to decide how I feel about cosmetic surgery and Botox.

Even though this book is all about handling the emotional side of the menopause, I had thought I would end up taking a stand one way or the other: either grow old gracefully and let the experiences of life show on my face and body, or make adjustments with input from the medical community. For some women, this question is a no-brainer: their attitude is 'If I can afford it and I look better, why not?' For others, it is a question of simply accepting what they look like – and, of course, financially not everyone has the choice.

There is no right answer; there is just the solution that is right for you. Personally, at the moment I'm favouring the natural route and can't see myself deviating from that (but never say 'never'!) Besides, my mother looked pretty good at 80, so I'm hoping I've enough of her genes to get a similar result.

I was struck by something that a friend wrote to me on this topic. I had never thought of her as the sort of person who was self-obsessed or fanatical about how she looked. In her case, the menopause was brought on by chemotherapy. This is what she said:

'I hadn't appreciated what it would be like to grow old – and almost overnight. I look at my photos now and see a much older woman, wrinkled and tired. I thought people who bought creams and potions and took fish-oil supplements were stupid and those who had plastic surgery were crazy. Having experienced pain and helplessness, it was far worse than my imaginings and now I'm fighting time just like all the people I thought were silly. I have no intention of growing old gracefully. I have far too many body lotions, face creams, hair conditioners, smoothers and de-frizzers; I take five different tablets a day as well as my anti-oestrogens (some aid in warding off cancer, others try to compensate by boosting bone density and joint lubrication); I bought a load

of gym equipment so I can exercise a lot; I am contemplating plastic surgery to tidy up the smaller breast and reduce the other to a similar size. I wonder about a face-lift. Looking at myself from outside, I am a self-obsessed nut-case.'

In the end, you cannot really hide what is happening and you have to make your own decision for yourself about what approach you will take. I admire the women who do, and those who don't. It's also important to remember that beauty comes from the inside as well as the outside.

For me, the biggest change I notice is the texture of my skin. I remember vividly the first time I noticed the skin on my face was changing. It was early morning, I was sitting on a train heading into London and, as I bowed my head to read my book, I felt the tiniest pull of gravity on the skin of the lower part of my face and around my jaw-line. It was an infinitesimally small movement, but what a huge shock to me. That was probably six or seven years ago and it was one of the tiny signs that changes were on their way.

Ever since then, I find myself going about looking closely at the skin of other women, particularly those who I think are a similar age to myself, comparing it with my own. There it is: visible evidence that I am not alone but, simultaneously, I have gained a surprise entry to a sisterhood that was previously unavailable to me. It's wonderful, there is a closeness and a support for and from women of a certain age. It's hard to put your finger on but, as an example, it is when you get a knowing look, a smile of sympathy and support from a complete stranger who recognises what is going on when you start to take off gloves, coat, scarf on a chilly day on a cold tube train!

What you resist persists

I came across the phrase "What you resist persists" when I was on a spiritual course, I don't know who said it originally. Recently, I have seen it written with an extra phrase added on:

What you resist persists, what you accept changes

When you push something away from yourself, you still give it attention and energy. The more we focus on something – either negative or positive – the more likely we are to bring it into reality.

You might be familiar with my experience of this, I certainly know it's true when I am on a diet: the more I focus on not eating certain foods, the more I want to eat them. Paradoxical eh?

What about this one: I was going away on a special weekend with my sisters and our husbands, all together, for the very first time in my life. I was really looking forward to it, and desperately hoping that we would all be able to go and that no one would get ill or come down with a cold or a bug or anything like that. I consciously stayed away from anyone who was coughing, snuffling and sneezing. Then, on the Thursday before, I had a two-hour train journey on a packed train, sitting right next to a person with the worst cold in the world! Guess what? I woke up on Friday morning, our departure day, with a cold brewing that lasted the whole four days and really spoiled the experience. I was so ill I couldn't go shopping and *that* hardly *ever* happens! You might say that it's just coincidence; my view is that we get what we focus on. I would probably have done a lot better had I focused on keeping fit and healthy, rather than on not getting a cold.

I have come across many women who talk a great deal about the negatives when it comes to the menopause. I guess it is tempting to offload on others when we get an opportunity to actually talk to someone about it, since it is not the sort of thing that generally comes into day-to-day conversations. I know for myself, at times I do get frustrated and annoyed with how I feel about it, and I'll tend to exaggerate the symptoms; sometimes I do that just to illustrate the point, or sometimes to amuse others. The problem with this is that if I keep focusing and thinking about the negative, I am magnifying my experience of the negative just by the way I talk about it.

Mind your language

The language we use to describe things actually changes the reality. The words we choose can actually change how we experience things. Here's what I mean by that:

Imagine you are waiting for a bus with four friends, you've been at the stop for over 20 minutes, the bus comes along but it is full and does not stop. Here's how each of the friends might describe the experience:

Grumpy Gail:
I'm absolutely furious about this, this is ridiculous! How dare they run a rubbish bus service like this? It's a disgrace!

Irritated Iris:
I'm annoyed; this sort of thing really gets on my nerves and makes me cross.

Bothered Belinda:
I'm a bit miffed; usually the bus service is better than this. Oh well, I expect there will be another one soon.

Chilled Cheryl:

Oh well, never mind, at least we are not alone and it's not raining either ... I expect three buses will be along in a minute.

By describing the experience differently, each person has a different feeling about it. When we label an emotion, as in the examples above, we start to feel it as we have described it. In the first example, the person is furious and can easily wind herself up into a rage about it. In the final example, the person is philosophical about the situation and does not let it bother her at all.

The words you choose to describe what you feel will turn that feeling into the reality. By labelling an emotion negatively we turn a 'nothing' into a 'something'.

So, as an end to this chapter, here are a couple of little activities to do:

- Listen to what you say to yourself about the menopause, Pay attention to the type of language you use and your choice of words. What is the story you tell people?

- Ask yourself this question and reflect on it occasionally during today, tomorrow and perhaps for a whole week:

  "If this is a very special and precious time of my life, what can I learn and discover from it?"

- Ponder on this quote:

  Every day may not be good, but there's something good in every day
  (Author Unknown)

Chapter 3

Me and My Emotions

"Let's not forget that the little emotions are the great captains of our lives and we obey them without realizing it"

Vincent Van Gogh

Like me, I suspect you wish you did not have to deal with all this menopause stuff, but if it is here, let's make the best of it and handle it the best way we can.

We can deal with the physical symptoms with medicines, hormones, herbs and supplements if we want to; I call this the 'outside-in' approach. Or, instead of just focusing on an external solution, we can take the 'inside-out' approach. This is where we stop and look at internal solutions. I believe our state of mind is central and critical, not only to how we experience the menopause, but also to what we make of this time of our life.

Really, this book is all about managing your state of mind and your emotions, both for yourself and those around you. It aims to enable you to be aware of your moods and how you feel, giving practical techniques and strategies so that you have a choice of behaviours, not just the automatic or knee-jerk reactions.

Recently I was walking down the road and experienced a tiny urinary leak; my almost immediate automatic reaction was to get annoyed and upset and to say to myself something like, "Oh flip, another flipping symptom, that's all I need, my bladder to start playing up, I'll be needing those wretched 'lady-leak-pads' instead of sanitary protection". (I have to say, the language was a lot more colourful than I have described here!) I could have allowed that to ruin my day, but instead I caught myself and checked my thinking. In a few moments, I found a different way of looking at it. I reframed it like this, 'I expect this is a one-off because it's cold, but I'll take it as a sign to do something about it; pelvic floor exercises are definitely on the agenda from now on.'

The first comment frames the situation as a negative that I have to deal with and put up with; the second reframes it into something I can do something about. Both viewpoints are perhaps valid, but the most useful is the second one where I am in charge and have some control.

That was just a tiny example of how we can help ourselves by paying attention to what we think and feel, how we see the world and what we say to ourselves. Throughout the book you will find activities, techniques and tips to help you make small changes to make big things better. There are ways of thinking that will give you some new perspectives and there are lots of questions that you can ask yourself as you go along that will give you new insights into yourself and your situation.

There are several helpful and useful exercises to do, if you choose to. The more time you spend on this, the more you will learn about yourself. This book is not about me telling you how to think about the menopause and your life; it's about you discovering how you really think and feel deep down and working out for yourself the best way for you.

What I do say is:

    Attitude is key

    You get what you focus on

    You have a choice

Imagine how pleased you will be when you get to the other end of the menopausal journey knowing that you have made every effort to smooth the way for yourself. (Yes, there is the other end to the journey and there is light at the end of the tunnel that is not the train coming!) How delighted will you be when you emerge with your sense of self enhanced and your personal relationships improved? How will you feel when other women come to you and ask "How did you do it?" What might be your reply – that you focused on the positives? That you looked at it as a great learning experience about yourself? That you felt it was an adventure to be marvelled at? That you embraced life in spite of it, or that you grew and developed because of it?

Well, if you do not already have the answer, and even if you do, read on and find out more.

Emotions, feelings and moods

Feelings are our constant companions, they can sustain or sabotage us; if we acknowledge them and deal with them productively, our lives will be simpler and easier. They are like waves: an ever-varying, constant ebb and flow. There is no stopping them and they have energy of their own. You can choose which ones to ride, which to jump over and which to skip away from and return to. Your feelings are your own, created within you. No one else can make you feel anything without you allowing it.

I thought the menopause would bring a welcome end to the irrational mood swings and the negative emotions that used to accompany my periods. Hah! Not yet so for me, I'm afraid! It seems that the PMS I had still seems to be present, possibly renamed as 'pre-menopausal symptoms', perhaps to be replaced later by 'post-menopausal symptoms' with something-else-menopausal in between! Who knows? In the meantime, what I do know is that, every now and then, I get overwhelmed by feelings of anxiety, paranoia, irritability and sadness, to mention just a few! It comes from nowhere and so far I can't pinpoint a reason, it just arrives. When this happens, I'll sometimes say that if I were still having periods, then this is the week I would be having one!

There are times when I find it hard to recognise that it is a just a mood or a passing feeling that will be over soon, dealing with it as such, and not allowing it to overtake my whole afternoon/day/life! These emotions, feelings and moods can be harder to handle than the physical symptoms, especially since the emotion colours how I see the situation and how I react.

What a fabulous sense of timing nature has! Just at the moment when we want to kick back and enjoy ourselves – Wallop! Here's something else to deal with. Many women are already coping with challenging situations: aging parents, children leaving home, the empty nest syndrome, living with grumpy teenagers, children approaching puberty, the final decision on whether to have a child, or even some with newborns. Any of that's enough to send you doolally, never mind the unwelcome menopause symptoms!

Feelings, emotions, moods – on a page, these words can look fairly innocuous. From an intellectual perspective, we can nod and say, "Oh yes, I know what that means," and accept that they are part of a person's make-up. However, when they occur in reality and we actually experience them, it is a different story. They can blind us to reality, cause us to say things we don't mean, make us treat the people around us with cruelty and disdain, trigger rude or bad behaviour towards others, or they can cause us to withdraw, to turn in on ourselves and shut out everyone else. Emotions and feelings can have a serious effect – not only on the person experiencing the emotion, but also on the people around them.

That is the reason for writing this book. I believe that if we can recognise, accept and work with our emotions, then the menopause transition will be an easier passage. There are many useful tools and techniques to help us; in this book I'll share several that I know are helpful; that way you can choose the ones that work for you.

Why is it important to handle the emotional side?

Because emotions colour everything, they grab us and hold us in a tight grip, they whisper untruths of doubt and negativity, and they sometimes show us a narrow and biased view of reality. Obviously it is not our positive emotions I am talking about here, I'll take as many of those as I can get! I'm referring to things like mood swings, negative emotions, emotional outbursts: feelings and reactions that seem to come from nowhere and knock us off balance. They can be upsetting and bewildering. Some of us let fly and some of us turn inwards. I know I hate it when I feel sad and depressed for no particular reason, or when I realise subsequently that I have been completely unreasonable. One male friend described living with his wife as 'A b****y nightmare. She's vile to me, bursts into tears at the drop of a hat for no apparent reason, then the next day she says nothing about it, there's just a big blanket of silence. I don't know if I can take it any more'.

Anxiety, mood swings, tiredness, irritability – all possible symptoms of the menopause. Wouldn't it be great to get some control over these to help ease your way? Not only to make your life easier, but to prevent hurt and damage to those around you. A friend shared the following story:

Sarah was a sunny child, happy and cheerful. Brenda, her mother, began showing some emotional symptoms of the menopause, often being irritable and impatient, just as Sarah was reaching 15. Brenda would frequently find fault and criticise her clothes, her make-up and her friends. Sarah felt as if she could not do anything right. She began to withdraw from her mother, she didn't tell her anything about her life outside the home or at school in case that drew more disapproval. Sarah's self-confidence started to suffer and she began to think that life was not worth living; she decided that she had to escape and left home at 16. Subsequently, she fell in with a 'bad crowd' though was lucky to have some good friends to help her get her life back on track.

Brenda was a strong and strict woman, and had no idea of the impact she was having on the life of her daughter. She did not know why her daughter was so distant with her, and did not have the communication skills to talk it through with her. They drifted further and further apart. They now see each other rarely and their relationship is fairly superficial. Brenda would love to see more of her daughter and would like to be more involved in her life, but Sarah is not so keen.

Neither of them knows what to do or how to resolve the situation.

In that scenario it was the emotions coming out: a little criticism here, a little disapproval there, on a fairly frequent basis, with the mother not really showing any love and affection, very possibly because she was caught up in her own emotional turmoil.

Of course it's not just the menopause that can cause our emotions to flare up. Tiredness can be a big factor, too. It's not only small children who get cross and grumpy at bedtime!

When you think about it, they way we feel affects everything in our lives. It affects our body, the way we hold ourselves, our facial expressions, even our heartbeat. It affects our mind because our thoughts are filtered, depending on how we feel; our enthusiasm and motivation are all generated by how we feel. It affects our inner self and our well-being. Our feelings can raise or drop our spirits.

Here is a story that I heard a while ago, about an older Cherokee man who is teaching his grandson about life.

"A fight is going on inside me," he says to the boy. "It is a terrible fight and it is between two wolves.

One is evil. He is anger, envy, sorrow, regret, greed, selfishness, arrogance, self pity, guilt, resentment, inferiority, lies, false pride, superiority and ego.

The other is good. He is love, joy, peace, hope, serenity, humility, kindness, benevolence, empathy, generosity, truth, compassion and faith.

This same fight is going on inside you and inside every other person."

The grandson thinks about it for a minute and then asks his grandfather, "Which wolf will win?"

The old Cherokee replies, "The one you feed."

We get what we focus on. So be sure you are paying attention to what you want and not what you don't want.

The Grief Cycle

I want to talk about this because it helps to see the menopause as part of a process and that there are normal phases that we go through. Some people sail through the menopause with barely a symptom, whilst others struggle – not only with how their body is behaving, but also because they feel different and experience unwanted negative emotions such as anger, irritability and sadness.

Some of those emotions are about the loss of what you once were: that young, dynamic person with the lovely youthful skin and body. Now the years have gone past and it is time to **mourn who you once were**. It's definitely worth taking some time to think over the **grief cycle** (Elisabeth Kübler Ross). Her work was on grief and bereavement, though it also applies in other highly stressful situations in life such as dealing with change, redundancy or illness. When we think about the menopausal stage of our lives and the loss of our younger self, this cycle applies here too. There are five stages in the cycle.

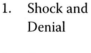

1. Shock and Denial

2. Anger

3. Bargaining

4. Depression

5. Acceptance

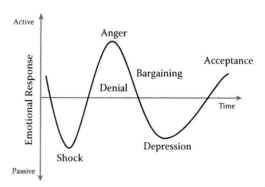

The cycle is not a progressive set of steps that arrive one after the other in a timely manner; it's more of a framework to help us understand the process. Some steps can pass very quickly, steps can be missed out; it's not always a forward progression and some people might get stuck at a particular step. Some people in some situations can go through the stages very quickly, in half an hour or less, others can take years. It's helpful to understand the process and notice where you are in it so that you can accept it, do something about it yourself or get some help from someone else. Here are the stages in more detail:

The Grief Cycle

Stage 1	Shock and Denial	Once we have started breathing again after the initial shock, we refuse to recognise or accept the situation or what is happening. We avoid the issue and pretend it's not happening.
		'This can't possibly be happening to me, I'm too young, I'm only 48 (or 50, 52, whatever age)'
		'I'm not having this!'
		'Gosh I've not had a period for a while, I must be pregnant!'
Stage 2	Anger/ Emotion	The emotions kick in. We want someone to blame. We can be angry with ourselves or with the people around us. Often we are not rational. I was furious that the decision on whether or not to have children had been taken away from me. Then I became really sad about it. I was mourning the child that I would never have.
		'How dare you make this happen to me!'

Stage 3	Bargaining	Initial shock and emotions have calmed down, then we start looking for some way round the situation. Trying to get our own way, bargaining with whatever higher power we believe in. 'There must be something I can do ...? Please ...'
Stage 4	Depression	The person recognises the inevitable, they focus on the negatives and become deeply despondent. Sometimes they turn in on themselves, avoiding the world. Viewing themselves as a victim of circumstances, they have feelings of hopelessness and helplessness. 'Poor Me, it's not fair.' 'I can't help it, it's not my fault.' 'I'm going to bed for six months and hiding under the covers.'
Stage 5	Acceptance	The person has tried all the avoidance tactics and realises that what they are doing is not working and that they need to get some control back and take action. They accept the situation and begin to deal with it in a more positive and forward-looking way. 'I am where I am, what am I going to do about it?' 'Nobody can do anything about this but me, best I do something.'

When you look at this grief cycle, and think about other instances of grief, can you recognise the stages from those other experiences?

Now you can take a moment to think about your own menopausal journey. Which stage are you at? Or perhaps you can recognise this from someone else's behaviour.

Here is a little more detail about each of the stages:

Stage 1 - Shock and Denial

I'm thinking that someone who was either in shock or denial might not be reading this book. They might be paralysed by fear or busy looking the other way, being very busy, occupying their mind with other things in order to ignore the symptoms or the evidence. At this point, we either can't really think about it clearly, or we don't want to see reality. The objective is to kick-start your thinking and start to deal with it bit by bit. It can be really overwhelming, frightening and upsetting to realise that the time has come and the symptoms of the menopause are appearing.

Things to do – the idea is to get your brain moving on this one, so I recommend:

- Starting to write your feelings in your journal. How you feel will vary from day to day and it will be useful for you to be able to look back on what you have written and get some perspective

- Actively seek out people you can talk to about this – family members or friends

Janet said she did not like to talk to friends in case they were not at the same stage as her. She was with a group of friends and had broached the topic of thinning hair. They all looked at her blankly and seemed to have no idea what she was talking about. She was worried that it would cause a distance in their friendship. So choose carefully who you want to discuss it with.

Stage 2 - Anger

The problem with anger is that when we are angry, we can't think straight. When we are angry, our nervous system, mind and body, are in the state of Fight or Flight. As human beings, this is our basic survival response. It is a biological reaction over which we have no control. Our brain senses danger and the body reacts immediately with the intention of saving us, so we get a shot of adrenaline, our heart rate and breathing rate speed up and blood which would normally go to the brain is diverted to our limbs to enable us to fight or run away. I met a surgeon once who told me that when we are in this state, it is like we have had a pre-frontal lobotomy – we are unable to think correctly because that part of the brain has almost closed down. (Note, I am not a neuroscientist but I know intuitively, as you do, that this is how it feels.)

Here are four ways to help you avoid letting anger get the better of you:

1. Choose not to react from a place of anger. Decide to control the emotion and stay in control.

2. Stop and count to ten. This is simple but it really works. Just focus on the numbers and think of nothing else. It will take you out of the emotion and then you can decide what to do or say next. Or try counting down from 10, relaxing as you go

3. Control your state. Breathe in for two counts and out for four counts – keep doing this for a minute or so. The brain realises that the Fight/Flight response is not required because you have control of your breathing. So it then turns off what I call 'red alert mode'.

4. Disassociate yourself from the situation. Imagine that you can step or float out of your body and watch yourself and your behaviour. See the emotion you are displaying and, from this perspective, think about what actions you can take to improve the situation.

Stage 3 - Bargaining

At this stage we are on the road to acceptance, but this is a fruitless activity which does not move us forward. The relentless passage of time wins and no amount of bargaining will stop or reverse the process. This might not be a phase that lasts long, but the sooner you get past it the better.

Stage 4 - Depression

It's not surprising that women might feel depressed at this time of life: body changes, the end of the reproductive years, hot flushes, night sweats and, for some, children leaving home and the empty nest syndrome. Really, even a saint might find it hard going. You could even say it would be abnormal not to feel stressed with all that going on!

The research on it is inconclusive as to why it happens, and not all women get depressed. If it persists, though, get some professional help, go and see someone who has the expertise to help you. The obvious choice would be your doctor, but you could also consider homeopathy or therapy.

Stage 5 - Acceptance

Hallelujah! I have seen the light! I accept this new self and I'm looking forward to the future! This is the bit that is worth waiting for and, in fact, according to the Jubilee Report (which compares menopausal women now compared to 50 years ago)

65 per cent said that they were personally happier now than they had been before the onset of their menopause.

The best part of this phase is thinking and planning what you are going to do next and learning more about this fabulous person you are now becoming. (There is more about this in Chapter 10 which is about Taking Charge).

Irritability

Being irritable is something that everyone feels from time to time, not just women going through the menopause. However, many menopausal women say that they feel more irritated.

You really don't need me to tell you that being annoyed and irritated is a horrible feeling, and showing that emotion to others can be very destructive. Sometimes we get cross and snappy with people, especially our nearest and dearest, and even though we know we should just keep quiet, we 'have a go' just the same. As I look back, I can't remember one single time when I was justified in behaving this way, or any time when it was the right way to behave and got me the result I wanted. All that happens is that everyone who is involved gets stressed and the situation is made worse.

Here are some things that you can do to help you through those moments:

First of all, remove yourself from the situation, just go somewhere else where you can stop and think. Anywhere will do: garden, kitchen, living room, bathroom, hallway, outside, anywhere as long as you are not where you were! Just the fact of removing yourself will change your state and will stop you from creating havoc. Also, from there you can look at the situation dispassionately.

Control and slow your breathing. Breathe in and out slowly, as you count to ten.

Identify what are your triggers, what sets you off?

Notice if you get any physical pre-warning; for example, one lady said she felt heat at the back of her neck so she knew her anger was coming.

Walk away – mid sentence if you need to, take a pause and think about what you really want to say and what message you really want to get across (thereby avoiding the response from the others of 'oh no, here she goes again'!)

Tell others how you feel, calmly, so that they can have a chance to work out how to react. Just by saying, "I feel really grumpy and annoyed today," gives them the opportunity to at least give you a wide berth.

Ask yourself what is really going on. Are you really mad with them or is it something inside of you that you are avoiding, or perhaps you just need to give yourself space.

Take responsibility, do something about it, remember that even a tiny shift in your behaviour can change everything. And you know, just being aware of what you are doing and how you are behaving will help you to deal with it.

Ask yourself, 'Will this really matter in an hour, a week, a month, a year?' If the answer is 'yes' then far better to think about how you are going to say it; if the answer is 'no', then consider holding your tongue, save your breath for something that matters.

Find a specific place in the house where you go to have these conversations or rants, so that every room is not contaminated by having had an argument take place in it.

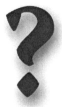 Question: when you are in a rage, if someone offered you £1,000,000 to stop and be calm and pleasant, would you be able to do it? If the answer is 'yes', that means you have control over the outbursts.

As you know, the mood passes but the aftermath can be permanent.

Ask yourself these questions:

- Does this need to be said, will it help the situation?

- Does it need to be said by me?

- Does it need to be said now?

If the answer to any of these questions is 'no', then leave it alone; take control of yourself and just don't go there. Why? Because in the short term you might achieve something like venting your feelings or saying something that you feel you need to say. Whilst this might make **you** feel better, it's important to recognise and remember that, in the long term, if you continue with that destructive behaviour, it will cause the erosion of the relationship. What I have learned is this:

There will always be a right time to say what you want to say

Besides, other people usually react badly by being spoken to by someone who is irritable. Wait until you feel better disposed towards them. In the meantime, work out how you can get your message across in a way that shows them respect and is non-emotional. It is also really helpful if you let go of blame or judgement of the other person. They are fine as they are and they are probably just doing their best; stop making them wrong. Look instead for a solution to the problem.

Technique: Freeze Frame

A fantastic technique devised by the HeartMath Institute to help reduce stress. When we are irritated, we are definitely stressed. It works by helping us control the Fight/Flight response with our breathing. (The Fight/Flight response is the automatic human survival mechanism that enables us to run away fast, or stay and fight if we find ourselves in a life-threatening situation.)

Here are the five steps of this process.

1. Recognise the feeling and FREEZE-FRAME it, take a time-out. This means pausing like you would pause a video recording as soon as you notice the negative emotion and/or the stress. (this isn't always so easy, either because you are caught up in the emotion or because you don't think - you are just acting in automatic. For example, if someone is really getting on your nerves or irritating you, it might be your habit to tell them straight or get them to stop doing what they are doing.)

2. Focus on the area around your heart, pretend you are breathing through your heart; keep your focus there for ten seconds or more. (Shift your attention away from your head and your thoughts.)

3. Recall a positive fun feeling or time you've had in your life and try to re-experience it. (Thinking about something positive changes your state of mind and that changes how you feel.)

4. Now using your intuition, common sense and sincerity, ask your heart what would be a more efficient response to the situation, one that would minimise future stress.

5. Listen to what your heart says in answer to your question. (This is an effective way to stop those automatic thoughts and emotions and find your own common-sense solution.)

Fear – an emotion almost worthy of a chapter to itself!

Whenever we take a chance and enter unfamiliar territory or put ourselves into the world in a new way, we experience fear. Very often this fear keeps us from moving ahead with our lives.

The trick is to FEEL THE FEAR AND DO IT ANYWAY
Susan Jeffers

The menopause delivers us into this unknown territory and puts us in a landscape which was familiar and is now changed by a new perspective. At a time in our lives when we were expecting things to be easier and more settled – Wham! Here comes something completely new to get to grips with. And, what's more, everyone experiences it differently, so you can't just follow the recipe of how to deal with it. It seems that, in order to handle it effectively, we have to find solutions and learn about ourselves all over again.

I would add that this episode of learning about myself is a LOT easier than the self-discovery that I experienced during my teenage years. What a nightmare that was! Lack of self-esteem, self-confidence problems, paranoia about the world, unfamiliar territory, emotions all over the place, moody, nobody understood me. Wait a minute! Isn't that the same as this? Hah! Who would have thought, eh? Whilst I'm being a bit tongue in cheek about this, it's also useful to note that you have experienced this sort of thing before, in a different context, but nevertheless a similar sort of thing.

I've seen the word fear turned into a mnemonic:

FEAR = False Expectations Appearing Real

We are brilliant at creating disaster scenarios in our heads about things that might or could happen. In one sense, this is quite useful to us because it helps us to view how a situation might play out; we create multiple scenarios, and then choose the one that works best. This enables us to evaluate what might happen and to spot any problems so that we can refine the actions we might take.

However, sometimes we forget that these are just imagined versions of events, not the real thing. In fact, if any one of us were able to predict the future accurately by imagining what might happen, and then for that prediction to actually happen in the real world, it would be nothing short of a miracle; and what's more it would earn you a fortune. So, in the meantime, before you make your millions by correctly guessing /predicting the future, here is another way of looking at it.

FEAR = Forgetting Everything is All Right

When you are creating your scenarios, make sure you also remember to imagine the versions where everything turns out just fine. In fact, in most situations our fears are unfounded. I know that some people will have been in some terrible situations, but we can, and do, get over these things; we learn to live with them, and often we are stronger for it. In fact, it is from those experiences that we develop and grow and find out more about ourselves. It is in our darkest hours that we discover deeper qualities and abilities and, once we have found out what there is to learn from those situations, we can begin to leave them behind as part of our lessons in life.

Here's what a friend of mine said about fear:

'If you touch on naked fear in your book ... I've spent the last year or so trying to get pregnant and thought that my husband's youth might compensate for any age issues with my body, but now I feel I've gone from one extreme to another and that I'm staring down the abyss of the menopause and never having children! Luckily it's never been a huge issue for me, although I think it will be for him, but I'm really struck by the polarity of my situation and the appalling lack of control which I really hate!'

So what fears might we have? For example:

Fear of
Lack of control
Change
The unknown
Losing who I once was
Death
Old age
Loneliness
Losing friends

A dear friend sent me this, and I think it is the most wonderful resource to help us through scary, difficult or challenging times, it's called Two Days.

TWO DAYS

There are two days in every week about which we should not worry, two days that should be kept from fear and apprehension. One of these days is yesterday, with its mistakes and cares, its faults and blunders, its aches and pains. Yesterday has passed forever beyond our control. All the money in the world cannot bring back yesterday. We cannot undo a single act we performed. We cannot erase a single word we said. Yesterday has gone forever.

The other day we should not worry about is tomorrow with its possible adversities, its burdens, its large promise and perhaps its poor performance. Tomorrow is also beyond our immediate control. Tomorrow's sun will rise either in splendour or behind a mask of clouds, but it will rise. Until it does, we have no stake in tomorrow, for it is as yet unborn.

That leaves only one day – today. Anyone can fight the battle of just one day. It is only when you and I add the burden of those two awful eternities – yesterday and tomorrow – that we break down. It is not the experience of today that drives us mad. It is the remorse or bitterness for something that happened yesterday or the dread of what tomorrow might bring.

Let us therefore do our best to live but one day at a time.

It's not the fear that is the problem; it is how we deal with it. I really expected that at this age, at this stage of my life, I would be in control, knowing how life worked; I would have got life sussed and everything would get easier. Hah! Isn't it funny how, as soon as we feel smug and self-satisfied, life has a way of side-swiping us with something to wipe the smile off our face. Even as I write these words, I'm thinking 'Barbara, you should be looking at this from a more positive angle'. Yes, that's quite true, particularly as I'll be talking about the menopause and positives later in the book. But I also think it's a good idea to have a balance, to see both sides of things and, after having done that, *then* err on the side of positivity.

Just before the menopause started, my life was pretty settled. I wasn't particularly happy, but it was OK, it was good enough. I was comfortable with where I was, I had a nice life and it felt pretty sorted. I wasn't really used to things changing, nor was I open to change because I was scared of what might happen. When my periods stopped and I realised that I was menopausal, it was like I'd been hit by a train. What a shock. In one fell swoop, everything I knew about my life was no longer solid.

Now, you might say that I was stupid not to expect it, given that I was about 48, but because I really only felt as if I was about 42, I was on quite a different wavelength.

I remember being in the company of friends who were talking about the menopause, hot flushes, and not sleeping ... and I was a million miles away, not listening, half thinking about other things because, of course, this wasn't going to be happening to me, not for at least another ten years. It was almost as if I had stuck my fingers in my ears singing La La La, La La to myself.

Six months after that, my periods stopped for four months, there was no way I could be pregnant, and the penny dropped. It wasn't the central heating coming on too early that was making me hot in bed. As I thought about it, the small symptoms, which had been invisible to me up until then, began to crystallise in my mind. All the fears that I mentioned earlier began to run riot in my head. I used my journal to get the thoughts out of my head, getting them on to paper seemed to minimise them. Through those writings I began to organise my thoughts and get some perspective on the situation, then I started to find out more about what to expect. The one thing that I came to realise during that reflection phase was this: I could either be scared and do nothing, or I could be scared and keep going.

A story from childhood springs to mind, which may be familiar to you. When I was learning to ride a bike – do you remember that feeling where someone grown-up is holding the saddle and you are pedalling along, confident that they are keeping you upright? Unnoticed by you, they let go of the bike and release you. After a little while, you realise you are, and have been, balancing all by yourself. Then, as you stop paying attention to what you are doing so that you can marvel at the magic, the grown-up shouts, "KEEP PEDALLING"!

Well, right now I just keep pedalling, a day a time.

As human beings, we have the most extraordinary ability to cope with adversity, challenges and dangers. We adapt, we create, we invent, we act. We do what it takes. That song *When The Going Gets Tough, The Tough Get Going* is absolutely true; inside we are all tough and actually we are tougher than we think we are. We'd have to be, to last this long in this mad world we live in!

So, just keep pedalling!

Browse back through the chapter and take a few minutes to ponder on the key points, learnings or discoveries for yourself from this chapter.

Is there anything that you will do differently?

Chapter 4

Taking care of your Relationships

"Whenever you're in conflict with someone, there is one factor that can make the difference between damaging your relationship and deepening it. That factor is attitude."

William James

Our relationships are so important in our lives, even though, at times, we just want to hide away under the duvet and have some peace and quiet for a while. Most of us need people around us. Sometimes we take our feelings out on other people, often the people who are closest to us. Some of the menopause symptoms such as irritability and anger, or even rage, seem to come from nowhere. Lashing out in anger without thinking about the other person is so damaging. If this is the case with you, be careful not to vent your frustration and let rip just because it's the menopause and that's how you feel, or because you think you can't help it. Whilst that release of emotion might make you feel better in the short term, in the long term it can ruin relationships. I was listening to a radio programme about the menopause recently and in the short space of the show, two men called in. They both said that their mothers were often in a bad mood, got angry, shouted a lot and criticised them constantly; that they felt they could not do anything right. It affected their whole relationship, they lost the closeness that they had with their mother and they never got it back. One said his mother turned into a monster when he was about 10. Even though you don't mean it to, it takes a terrible toll. Twenty or thirty years later, it still affected them enough to call a radio station about it.

I have a step-daughter. Early on, I used to get very frustrated with her; however, as she is not my child, I had to learn to bite my tongue and say nothing. I would go away and tidy my sock drawer and think carefully about how I was going to handle the situation and how I could get my point across and, at the same time, preserve the relationship. Sometimes I would write about it in my journal. These entries are illegible; even in my angry state, I wanted to make sure that no-one would ever read them! There are a few pages where I am so mad and I have pressed so hard with the pen that the page beneath is deeply marked by my words. Two years later, we have a fine relationship and I am so grateful that I did not let my emotions get the better of me.

Learn to stop and think. Your husband or partner, your children and your friends are so precious. They are constant, whilst your feelings are transitory. They deserve your respect; treat them well and take care of them (even if they are being irritating and not doing what you want them to do. Grrrr!)

The best way to handle it is to let people know. Tell them if you feel that your emotions are getting the better of you or own up if you realise you are being unreasonable. Then others can see that you are actually thinking about them. Use your brain, be clever about it, everyone is different and will need a different solution, but here are a couple of suggestions.

Three Chairs technique

This is a wonderful technique you can use to help you to see a situation from the other person's perspective. It is really useful when you are annoyed with them, you can't see why they are behaving in a particular way, or you just don't understand their point of view.

It sounds a little complicated to describe, but actually it is really simple. If you are thinking 'I'm not sure I can be bothered to do this', please give it a try. You will be amazed at the things you discover and come up with.

These are the steps and the instructions:

3 Chairs - Perceptual positions

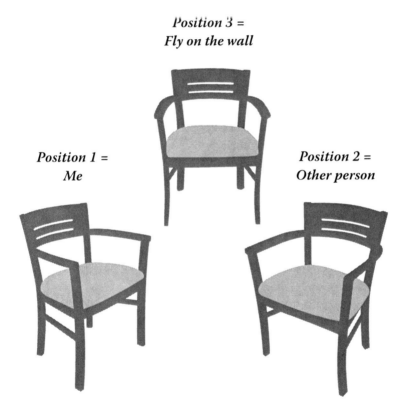

Position 3 =
Fly on the wall

Position 1 =
Me

Position 2 =
Other person

First, choose the relationship or situation you want to explore.

Take three chairs and arrange them in a triangle as if they were going to seat three people who are in conversation. It might be helpful to have someone else guide you through the instructions; otherwise you can make notes about what you learn/know at each position.

Decide which chair corresponds to which position. You are going to sit in each chair in turn. Don't just do this in your head. Shifting positions gives you new and different insights, so change chairs .

In Position 1, you are being yourself and seeing things from your own perspective.

In Position 2, you imagine you are the other person; pretend you have floated into their body; put yourself in their shoes; sit, act and speak as if you were them.

In Position 3, you become a 'fly on the wall'. Imagine that you are above and a little bit away, looking down on both the people in the chairs and in the situation.

The process is to sit in each chair and see things from that particular perspective and ask yourself the questions outlined below. The objective is to explore the situation from each perspective.

Start at Position 1, then move to Position 2, then to Position 3. Finally, return to Position 1 and notice what you have learned that is new and different.

Some people think, before they start this process, that it is a bit weird, that they will not find it easy, and can't see how they could get something out of doing the activity. It's worth giving it a go; try it and see what happens. Most people, once they get the hang of this, find it to be an invaluable tool that they can use in both their personal and professional life.

Advice: it's not enough just to do it in your head, you have to physically sit in each of the chairs and move positions to get the most out of this technique. You can either do it now, or make a note in your diary of when you will do it.

1st Position. Think about the situation, first from your point of view:

(I'm Barbara, and I'm looking at my relationship with John)

- How are things at the moment?

- What makes it difficult? What makes it easy?

- What are you thinking and feeling about this relationship or about the other person?

- What emotions are you experiencing?

Now leave your own viewpoint and prepare to look at the situation from the other person's point of view.

2nd Position. Now you become the other person; pretend to be that person, sit like them and speak as if you were them.

(Now I'm John, and I'm looking at Barbara who is sitting in chair Position 1)

- How are things from this perspective?

- What do you think and feel about?

- How do you see yourself in the relationship? How do you react?

When you have explored this, shake off that second position and move to sit in the chair of Position 3 'Fly on the Wall'.

3rd position. Consider both sides of the relationship dispassionately.

(I'm a 'fly on the wall' and I'm looking at Barbara and John)

- How are things from this perspective?

- What sort of relationship is it?

- What do you think of yourself (the one in Position 1) in this situation?

- How could this relationship or situation be improved?

Return to Position 1

Having looked at the situation from all three perspectives, return to sit in Position 1, review what you have learned and discovered about the situation.

- What is new and different?

- How can you improve the relationship?

- What will you do differently now?

You can use the three chairs technique in a number of situations, for example:

1. To help you prepare for a difficult conversation that you want to have with someone.

2. To enable you to explore a relationship that is not going very well.

3. To see things from another person's point of view.

I have used this with many coaching clients to help them think through the situation with their colleagues. I've used it to work out how to have a difficult conversation with my stepdaughter, my husband and my ex.

A friend of mine used it to work out how to ask her boss for a salary increase. Doing the exercise gave her a whole new perspective. She discovered that her boss thought she was a bit wet, that she lacked drive and commitment. As a result, she completely altered how she approached the situation. When she put her case forward subsequently, she was more direct and clear in what she wanted, with much less waffle than usual. Her straightforward and no-nonsense approach was successful: she got the raise!

It gets easier every time you practise, and even if you only discover one thing that you hadn't realised before, then it is worth the effort. You'll probably find that the more you engage your imagination, the more you'll get out of this activity.

(Note: some people say, "Well, I can't do this, because I can't possibly know what the other person is thinking". Whilst you are quite right, you cannot really know what is going on in their mind, but really that does not matter. What does matter is that you get a different way of looking at things that is usually unlike anything you have thought of before. The process still helps and gives you a way to see the situation from a different viewpoint, and having that new perspective will enable you to think differently about it. This often means that you have more choices of how to approach the situation.)

Reflect and Review

This time of your life, when things seem to be in a state of flux, is an excellent time to stop and think about how your main relationship is going; by that I mean with your partner, husband or significant other. Even if you are not in a relationship, the questions are still relevant. Give yourself some time – one or two hours – when you can sit comfortably in peace and reflect. The whole point is to think about how your life is going so as to identify if/where you want to make changes.

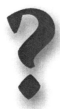 Some questions to ask yourself are:

- Am I happy with how things are?

- What, if anything, would I like to change?

- What can I do about the things that need to be changed?

Be really honest with yourself. There is no point pretending everything is fine if it isn't. Given that you might be only half-way through your life, or less, it is too soon to give up and accept mediocrity, there is so much more to come.

As you think about this, here are some things to look out for

- Have you lost the sense of yourself as an individual, existing more as part of a couple?

- Do you sometimes take each other for granted?

- Do you feel that there are things you would like to change, but don't have the guts, or energy or skills, to broach the topic?

- Are you too busy or preoccupied to take time to focus on each other?

- How have you *both* changed over the last one, three or five years?

- Have you remembered to be grateful for what you have?

- What habits might you have developed that get in the way of you making the most of your life together? (e.g. putting off going somewhere special, or watching too much TV)

- Do you find it easy to criticise or be negative and forget about all the qualities and good points?

This is not a definitive list, but rather some suggestions you can think about. The menopause may throw up some changes in perspective for you. The purpose is to look at your relationship, how it works and how you feel about it, from a non-judgemental and objective perspective. Having reviewed the situation, you can then decide what you are going to do about it. The secret is to take responsibility and take action. There is no point in sitting back and waiting for things to improve by themselves, or hoping that someone or something else will happen that will move things along. You can make a difference for yourself.

13 Relationship Enhancers

If you would like to take your relationship to a new level, here is a *smorgasbord* of things you might to do improve it. Some you might love, others might be inappropriate for you. Choose the ones that will work for you, those that appeal the most and, if you feel inspired to have an even better relationship, invent some more that are not on the list.

1. **Renew:** find the things that you used to enjoy doing or experiencing, that you stopped doing, for whatever reason, and start incorporating them into your life again.

2. **Rekindle:** spice things up a little. Make time to flirt with each other, go on a date, add a little spice back into your life, seduce each other. Try finding small ways to increase the intimacy.

3. **Repair:** if there are things that have not gone well, say sorry if you need to, forgive each other and move on. Get things out into the open so that you can discuss them, resolve them and let them go.

4. **Release:** if the relationship is over, and it is time to move on, then be adult about it. Sometimes it's nobody's fault; people change, situations change. Be brave.

5. **Rebuild:** if you want to stay together, then build your new life together, being open and honest about what you want. Forgive yourselves and each other and start afresh.

6. **Reflect:** if your relationship has been going along in automatic for a number of years, give yourself time to think about it, considering what you love about being with the other person and admitting what could be better.

7. **Rejoice**: everyone is magnificent. Take delight in the skills, abilities and qualities of each other. Remember what makes them particularly special to you ... and tell them about it.

8. **Rebel**: maybe it's time to break out and do something different for a change, just to see what happens!

9. **Re-jig**: notice where you can make minor improvements that will make a major difference.

10. **Resolve**: don't let the little things that niggle you carry on. Get them out in the open and find a solution for them. Look for a win-win for both of you.

11. **Rediscover:** how to love and support each other! Find each other all over again, as you see each other with new eyes and a new perspective.

12. **Remember**: you are both individuals in your own right, so check that you treat each other with respect.

13. **Reconnect:** with each other as separate people. It's easy to take each other for granted and to think of the other person as just the other half of a couple. Nurture each other as individuals as well as part of the pair.

I believe that we all deserve to be happy in our relationships. They may have their ups and downs and challenges to deal with but, overall, our nearest and dearest should make us feel loved, needed and cherished. By the same token, we should make them feel the same. Pause for a moment and check whether that is true for you; then you might consider what you can do to nurture it and keep it that way. If this is not the way your relationship feels, then the question is: What are you going to do about it?

Marion had experienced first-hand staying in a relationship when it was not really quite right. It was what might be described as a mediocre situation; she didn't know how to change it, she was scared to rock the boat and was not brave enough to do something about it. Then circumstances forced her to take stock, finally she decided she would be better off on her own, feeling OK about herself rather than feeling unloved and undesired. The moment she made that decision, even though it was scary, it felt as if a huge weight had been lifted from her shoulders. Then, six months later, she met a wonderful new man, the love of her life. A year and a half later, they were married and now they are working on living happily ever after.

From what I've seen in the relationships around me, and also what I have experienced myself, if we are not happy we should say so early on, rather than saying nothing and letting things drift or get out of hand. Sometimes we are scared of having these conversations , but isn't it better to have a talk now about something that is bothering you, rather than to experience the pain of separation later because no-one said anything?

I know it can be easy to take people for granted in our busy lives. However, at this transition time of your life, it's worth taking the time to see how you can not only preserve but also enhance what you have.

Most importantly, though, if you know that your hormones create havoc with your emotions, try to manage your behaviour and your reactions when you are around others so that you keep safe the people who are important to you. It might be easier to be in charge of those reactions when you are with acquaintances or strangers; however it's more critical to be in control with our nearest and dearest.

As you go through the book you will find a number of activities and reflections that will help you to deal with this – writing a journal is one of them. Writing down those thoughts and feelings allows you to get them out of your head without hurting others in the process.

Take a few moments now to ponder on what you have read and thought about the contents of this chapter. Look back and consider the important learning points for you.

Chapter 5

Identity, Values and Beliefs

"There comes a point in many people's lives when they can no longer play the role they have chosen for themselves. When that happens, we are like actors finding that someone has changed the play."

Brian Moore

This chapter is an invitation for you to stop and think about *who* you are, what you believe and what is important to you.

Sometimes we are so busy doing our day-to-day activities, worrying about stuff and getting on with our everyday lives, that we don't have time to pay attention to ourselves. Over time, what we believe changes, what is important to us alters and our sense of identity shifts. The onset of the menopause is a time when our whole self feels as if it is in flux. When I look in the mirror, the face that looks back at me is the same face, and yet it is different. My body seems to be changing on a daily basis, and not for the better, either! A few more lines, changing skin texture, the odd hair on my chin, a little extra weight … and that's just on the outside. On the inside, I am experiencing a strange mix of self-confidence and self-doubt. It's time to stop and think about the fundamentals of inner life: Identity, Values and Beliefs.

By the way, this chapter is not designed to be the definitive work on Identity, Values and Beliefs. It is meant to help you to reflect and for you to take some practical action to think about you, yourself and your life, in the context of the menopause.

These are simple exercises to do, and they will give you many deeper insights into yourself.

Identity

As we go through life, our sense of self changes and morphs into something new at every stage: from childhood to our teenage years, to twenties, thirties, forties and fifties and beyond. Every decade brings us new learning and discoveries about ourselves. Everything that happens to us, everything we experience, makes us who we are and enriches us. As we know, our most trying times are those which make us the strongest: the times when we have been on the edge of failure and we have found our way through; or when we have made mistakes and learned from them; or when life has been hard for us but we have overcome the difficulties. I think of the menopause as one of these life-changing, character-forming types of challenge. Whilst it's not always so easy to handle, I know it will make me stronger. So, in a way I am looking forward, with some element of trepidation, to what there is to learn from this time of life. I wonder who I will be? Who will I become? What will I find in myself that I did not previously know about? Who do I want to be from here on?

I went to a conference recently and, on the way home, struck up a conversation with a fellow attendee about identity and the menopause. One view that she held was that our identity is rooted in our femininity, how we look, our attractiveness to the opposite sex and our ability to bear children. It seems to me that, once the menopause strikes, all those erstwhile important factors seem to fade into the distance, leaving me with the thought that I need to redefine 'ME'. The 'Old Me', or rather 'Previous Other Me' was great, but that is now passing and will be over soon and I need a new way of thinking about myself and *how* and *who* I will be in this new territory, this familiar and yet unfamiliar landscape.

Sue told me she felt bewildered, because all of a sudden the things that she did which used to get results, like flirting, smiling and batting her eyelashes to get her own way, stopped working overnight!

It's definitely worth taking some time to reflect on your sense of identity, stopping and thinking about who you are now and also who and what you are becoming. Here are a couple of activities that will help you to do that.

Activity: Who am I?

1.   **I am …**

There is a television commercial for a telephone company that suggests that we are everyone who we have come across in our lives who has inspired us. You can do this yourself; it's a lovely heart-warming exercise to do, adding people who have helped and supported you, special people who add something to your existence. Why not give it a go and see who comes to mind and for what reason? Here is the start of mine:

I am my mother who taught me to aim higher

I am the people I coach who inspire me by their action and progress

I am my friends who accept me for who I am

I am Tim who told me I was smart and believed in me

I am my husband who loves and supports me through everything

And so on. Try it for yourself, just think about whose influence has been valuable in your life and start the sentence with

I am …

Another way of looking at the identity question is to look at it from the perspective of roles: I am a daughter, a sister, a dog owner, a wife and so on. The easiest way of doing this is by using a mind map; instructions on how to do this follow.

Technique

Making a Mind Map

Mind-mapping is a terrific technique; it is the brainchild of Tony Buzan. It gives you a simple and easy way to capture ideas, order your thinking and also to be creative, using the way our brain works. Often when we are thinking about things, we will put them in lists, but our brain works in a more organic way: it thinks about something for a little while, gives us some ideas, then jumps to a new idea and then might jump back to the original thought, and so on. Mind maps involve putting the topic in the middle and then making the words radiate out from it on branches, like a spider diagram.

Here's how to do it:

- You will need coloured pens - fine-tipped felt pens are ideal - and a blank piece of unlined paper, A4 or larger

- Use the paper in landscape orientation

- In the centre of the paper, write the topic about which you want to think/write, surround it by a shape - for example a cloud

- Then, for each idea, draw a branch and print the idea on it in capitals. The length of the branch matches the length of the word. Use one word per branch. Branches should be thicker next to the main topic. You can then have branches that come off each branch

- Use at least three colours because it is attractive and stimulates our imagination and the right side of the brain

- It does not have to look perfect; it's just for you to help you think. So go ahead, play with it and enjoy yourself

So, now you know how to mind-map, take 15 minutes for a 'time-for-me' pause and think about yourself: who you are, your identity and create a mind map of that (you could also add who you were, in a different colour). I have not included a sample here because I would like you to really give yourself a free rein to do this in any way you like.

You might be thinking:

- I'll do that later

- I've not done this before, I'm not sure about this

- I can't really be bothered

- This isn't my kind of thing

My sister's comment on this was, "This is not something I would find easy to do. Lack of confidence or ideas for me would make this difficult, but sometimes when you are forced into a situation where you have to think it through, the ideas DO come."

Your mind map doesn't have to be perfect or look good or be anything other than a way of helping you think about something. You could even throw it away or burn it when you have finished it if you want to.

Remember, you are reading this because you want some new ideas, and that takes thinking time. Those new ideas will begin to be generated by what I have written here, but you can make them develop and expand and grow even more as you put your mind to them.

It's easy – just get the pens and the paper, and maybe a glass of water, and begin.

By the way, if you really feel that mind-mapping is just not for you and you don't like it, my suggestion is to give it another go and see if you can find any value in it and then, if you still don't like it, you can use lists instead.

Values

Our values are things that are important to us, they drive our behaviour, they inform our decision-making, they are the reason we get out of bed in the morning to do something! Our values change over time and, at the change of life, it is likely that our values will shift again. So it will be useful and interesting to see what our current values are and also see new values emerging.

We have an overriding set of values that we can call 'values for life'. To find out what they are, the question to ask is, 'What's important to me in my life?' Typical answers will be things like Family, Health, Work, Home, Security, Integrity, Relationship, Friends, People, Challenge, Travel. These may be typical sorts of answers, though every person's list will be different, either in obvious or subtle ways. Then we will have some subsets of those, such as Values for Family, Values for Health and Fitness and so on. Then, for each of those areas or subsets, you can ask the same question:

'What's important to you about X?' (X stands for whichever value you are asking about)

You could also ask, 'What do you value about X?'

Typical answers for Health might be: fitness, strength, flexibility, feeling good, being agile, mind-body connection, longevity, preventing illness, energy. Again, this is not an exhaustive list.

We tend to gravitate towards people who hold similar value sets to ourselves. We might think that our values are the same, and then occasionally we are shocked by the behaviour of a friend whose actions we think are quite unacceptable but, from their perspective, are absolutely fine. Here's an example. A friend of mine I have known for about 25 years called me to offer a great opportunity. "It's great," she said, "all you do is invest £3,000 and you will get £24,000 back. You just need to get another eight people to invest with you, and then they get eight people, and so on." From her perspective, it was brilliant; she'd get a great return on her investment. From my perspective, I was thinking about all the poor people at the bottom of the pyramid who would be out-of-pocket as and when the pyramid collapsed.

Similarly, we have all heard stories where a couple who have been living together happily for a long time decide to get married and then, a year after the wedding, they have split up and gone their separate ways. One explanation might be that their values for living together matched, but their values for marriage were at odds.

It's also worth mentioning that our values change over time, depending on age, circumstances and context. What is important to someone when they are eighteen, single, footloose and fancy-free, will be quite different from that same person's values 15 or 20 years later, when they are a successful businesswoman with a family, responsibilities a mortgage. Work-life balance would be significant to one person and completely irrelevant to the other. (I had no idea what work-life balance *was* until I was about 45!)

Discovering your own values

Time: one hour or more

Get a pen and paper - and by the way, don't even bother to read this if you are not going to do the activity - it's not something you can do in your head, and it takes a bit of reflection time.

This activity comes in several parts: the initial question is about your whole life, and the subsequent questions you can ask yourself about the different areas of your life. You should allow a couple of hours for this, although it doesn't need to be completed all in one go. You can do a bit at a time.

Part 1

Ask yourself the following question and write down what your answers are to it:

What's important to me in my life?

You might come up with three words, you might come up with 26 - that's quite all right.

When you think you have exhausted your responses, ask yourself the question again. Do this twice or three times more and add all your answers to your list.

Next, look through your answers and list them in order of importance with Number 1, the most important, at the top.

Hint 1:

If you are having trouble deciding between one item and another, here is how to sort out the more important one. Let's say you are trying to decide between Security and Health. You ask two questions:

Would it be all right if I could have Security and not Health?

Would it be all right if I could have Health and not Security?

You don't need to decide on one or the other, but you will find that one will feel and sound right to you over and above the other.

Hint 2:

Sometimes people say they find it hard to determine the correct order they go in. If that is the case for you, just do your best. What you come up with is not the one-time-only definitive list; remember these values change over time. You might also find that you need some time to reflect on some of the things that are on your list. And by the way, there are no right or wrong answers. This is your list, for you. You can change the contents of it if you want and you can change the ordering of it; just be truthful to yourself.

Now, focus on the top eight items on your list; those are the things that are most important to you and, what's more, those are the reasons why you do what you do. Stop for a few minutes and reflect on how your list of values is played out in everyday life.

Example:

One of my core values is helping people; in fact it is part of my identity, it's what I do. If I were sitting side-by-side on a train and in conversation with someone who told me about a problem they had, I would automatically want to help them. Work is also an important value for me, and writing this book, to me, is both work and helping people at the same time. Every morning, I get up early to do my writing; it is the most important part of my work at the moment. I have made a sort of rule for myself that I don't do anything else until I have done my writing. One morning, I received an email from my sister, asking me for help to write an important letter in relation to the health of our mother. I didn't even stop to think about it, but spent over an hour working on the letter before I even started my book-writing. Up until that moment, I hadn't realised that helping a family member was higher in importance than helping others. Now, you might say that it is obvious that I would think like that, but it wasn't, not to me, before that moment. When you do this exercise, you just don't know what you will discover about yourself and how you behave.

Part 2

Now you have discovered the eight most important areas of your life, you can follow the same process for each area, asking yourself the same questions, writing down your answers and putting them in order of preference.

Starting with your Number 1 value for life:

What is important to me about X?

Finally

Take some time to write in your journal about what you have learned and how it is useful to you.

Beliefs

Our beliefs, i.e. what we think is true, change over time; for example the existence of Santa Claus or the Tooth Fairy. Once, quite a long time ago I admit, I used to believe that they both existed ... and they still do! Just not in reality! Things we once believed were difficult are now just an easy, vague, faint memory, like learning to drive. What a trauma that was on the first day, and now it's second nature. Sometimes our beliefs become old and redundant without us noticing!

Our beliefs can either help us or hinder us. There are two main reasons for spending time thinking about this now: to identify beliefs that you currently have about yourself and also to explore what your beliefs are about this menopausal time. For example, do you believe it is a time to sit back, relax and let go, coasting gradually into the twilight years? Or do you believe it is a time to really change gear and go out and discover new people, things and places? You might have heard the old saying 'Life begins at forty' – well, I believe that fifty is the new forty!

I met a wonderful woman a few years ago whose mission in life was to help people improve their sight naturally without using spectacles. She was absolutely passionate about the techniques and the results she achieved. I think she was probably in her 40s at the time. I remember her saying to me that there was so much work for her to do, she would be at it for another 50 years! If you think about it, implicit in what she said is the belief that she will not only be alive at 90+, but also that she will still be working with people – a vocation she has a passion for. What an inspiration.

You've probably heard of the Pygmalion effect, also called the self-fulfilling prophecy, where whatever we *believe* is true actually *becomes reality*. Originally from Roman mythology, the story is about a sculptor called Pygmalion who created a statue of the perfect woman called Galatea. She was so beautiful he fell in love with her. He prayed to Venus, the goddess of love, to bring Galatea to life. His prayers were answered and they were united in love. George Bernard Shaw wrote a play by the same name about it, and there was also the film *My Fair Lady* starring Audrey Hepburn and Rex Harrison in which Professor Higgins believes that he can turn a flower girl into a Duchess, and he manages to achieve it.

The point of all this is that whatever we believe will happen is typically what ends up happening. Here's how the process works, illustrated by a small model I call the Belief Cycle

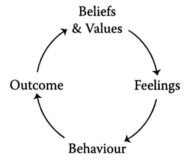

Our Beliefs and Values affect our feelings which, in turn, change how we behave, which influences the outcome which then confirms and validates our Beliefs and Values and so on.

The first time I saw this model, I was not particularly impressed with it; my thought was 'So what?' It all seemed to make sense at an intellectual level, but it didn't really grab me until something was said that made me see it in a new light. I was delivering a training course on assertiveness with a group of airline cabin crew. We were discussing this belief model and talking about how, in order to be assertive, you consider both your own rights as well as those of the other person. Depending on whether you believe you have a right to be assertive, or not, will determine whether you actually speak up for yourself and say what you want, or not. When a girl from the back of the group said, "Well it doesn't matter, because passengers think we are s**t anyway", I was completely stunned. As a former cabin crew member, that was a million miles away from my experience and what I believed.

Using this as an example, we can follow the model round to see how it works (we'll call this girl Mary).

Belief: Mary's belief is that passengers think badly of her, they don't respect her and they are dismissive of her.

Feelings: When she is at work, she feels angry, resentful and demotivated. (Would you want to serve people who think so badly of you?)

Behaviour: She is off-hand, cold and abrupt in her manner with passengers. She 'forgets' to do things people have asked of her. She isn't helpful and doesn't smile or talk to passengers.

(As you read this, you might perhaps recall being on the receiving end of someone who thinks and acts like her!)

Outcome: She does a poor job with the passengers who, as they are leaving the plane, walk past her and ignore her as if she isn't there. They say neither 'goodbye' nor 'thank you', they just get off. She then finds that her belief has been proved and reinforced, she has more evidence to prove herself right; in her eyes, passengers really do think she is 'sh*t'. Mary goes home miserable and fed up, wishing she had a different job.

We could also imagine that the next time she goes to work, the same thought patterns will probably repeat themselves and she might reinforce the belief even further.

Contrast this with the experience of one of her colleagues who believes that passengers think the cabin crew are wonderful (we'll call this girl Jane).

Belief: Jane's belief is that passengers think the world of her and her colleagues. She believes that they appreciate any effort she makes on their behalf and so goes out of her way to do a good job. She loves to go the extra mile for people because she loves to please them and see their gratitude.

Feelings: When she is at work, she feels happy, enthusiastic, motivated.

Behaviour: She is warm and friendly with the passengers. She smiles and likes to talk to people, find out more about them. She remembers to bring things that they have asked for, a glass of water here, a blanket there.

Outcome: Jane does a great job with the passengers and, when they get off, they smile, say 'goodbye', and 'thank you'. They also write in to say how much they appreciate her hard work. In her mind, this just goes to prove that she is right: passengers do think she is wonderful! Jane goes home, happy that she has done a good job and made people's journeys a better experience.

The funny thing is that Mary and Jane could have been working on the same flight, in the same cabin, with the same people and, because of their beliefs, Mary would get what she expected: negative passengers, and Jane would get what she expected: positive passengers.

That story talks about beliefs in relation to other people, but the same cycle also applies to the beliefs we hold about ourselves and our capabilities. Our own mindset colours and affects how we see the world. So remember, watch out what you believe in, because that is what you will make happen.

There is a great quote from Henry Ford on this topic: *Whether you think you can, or can't, you are right.*

So here's another illustration of how this model works, using one of my negative beliefs: 'I can't find time to go to the gym'.

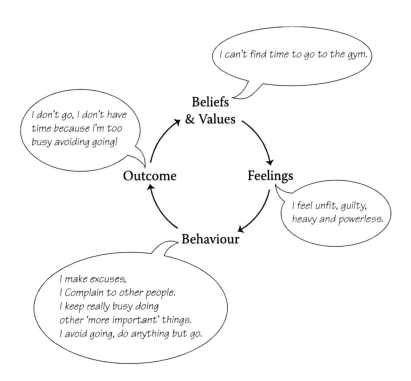

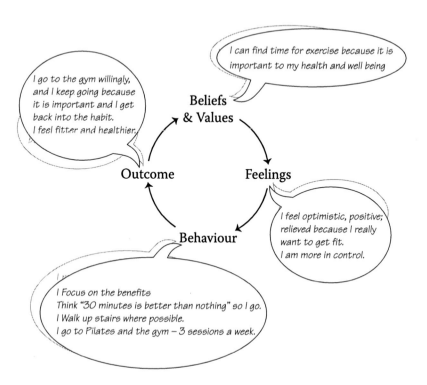

Activity – Unhelpful beliefs

Time: 20 minutes

Kit: Journal and two coloured pens and any paper, ideally A4 size

Part 1

Draw the Belief Cycle in the middle of the page. Then, with one of the coloured pens:

1. Write down a negative belief you hold about yourself, next to Belief on the model.

2. Next to Feelings jot down how you feel as a result of that belief.

3. Next to the word Behaviour, capture how you behave as a result of that belief and those feelings.

4. Finally, next to Outcome, note what the likely outcome would be as a result of your likely behaviour.

Part 2

Decide what would be a more useful or helpful belief. Using a different colour pen:

1. Write down the positive belief that you could choose to have, next to Belief on the model.

2. Next to Feelings jot down how you feel as a result of that positive belief.

3. Next to the word Behaviour, capture how you behave as a result of that new belief and those feelings.

4. Finally, next to Outcome, note what the new likely outcome would be as a result of your modified belief, feelings and behaviour.

Take five minutes or so to pause and think about what you have learned from this exercise.

When/if you have more time, take a belief about the menopause and repeat the exercise. There is an example below to illustrate.

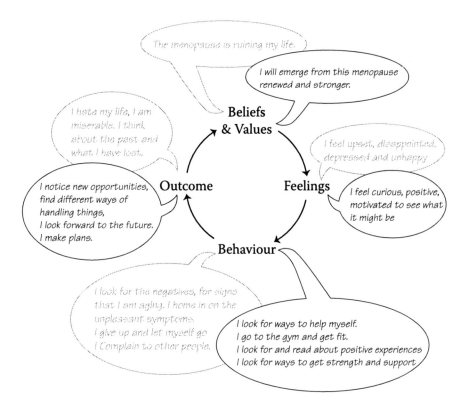

As you can see from the example above, what you think and believe has a direct impact on what you feel and how you behave, and that changes what happens in your life.

This model applies across our whole lives and is useful to help you see how you can rethink things to improve your world and the way you live.

Do you think the menopause is a nightmare with no end – or do you think it is an interesting and exciting time? Your choice, your outcome.

Have a care: if you think the world is full of badness, then that is what you look out for and notice and experience. Conversely, if you think the world is full of goodness, then it is. It all depends what you choose to focus on. If you take this thinking to its logical conclusion, then you need to be careful what you think about and what you wish for because that is what you will get. The question to ask yourself is 'What sort of world do I want to live in?' and then go looking for exactly that.

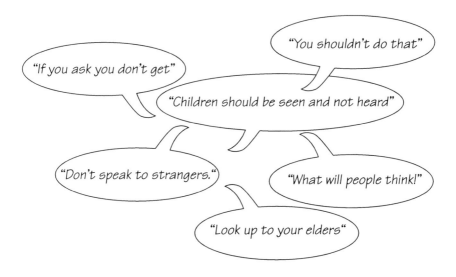

All these were messages that I got as a child. They were meant to help me to behave better, probably to make me easier to manage and also to keep me safe. The only problem with these sayings is that when they are repeated over and over again, they become a firm part of the belief structure about how life is. You will probably have a similar set of 'rules' that you heard as a child. Without realising it, these beliefs can still affect us years later in life.

Think about any of those old rules that you were given to live by. Some of them work really well, such as "you can do anything you want as long as you put your mind to it". Some are less helpful. I sometimes think that my quietness at dinner parties stems from that old mantra 'Children should be seen and not heard', followed quickly by 'What will people think? 'And so I keep quiet, and every so often someone else will say what I was going to say. And when that happens, I feel a fleeting sense of disappointment in myself. What a futile waste of energy, why didn't I just say what I was thinking in the first place and leave behind that insecurity and lack of conviction? Most of those rules are really of no use to me now in this menopausal state; why not just let them go?

Perhaps now is the time to leave all that behind, to step into your power and be all you can be, to stand up and be you, in all your glory. **You are magnificent!**

If, as you read this, you have doubts about the truth of the last statement, then think about it carefully. You can probably come up with many reasons as to why it is not true, but how many reasons can you think of to prove that it is true?

You are grown up now, you are in charge of your life and your destiny, and you can make things happen or not. You choose.

When we are at the change of life, it is perhaps time to revisit all those old beliefs and see if they still fit, as if we were taking them out of the wardrobe, having a good look at them, keeping the ones that work and throwing away the ones that don't.

What old, redundant beliefs might be holding you back from expressing yourself and doing what you want to do? Here's an activity to help you think about it.

Activity – Redundant beliefs and messages from childhood

Time: 15 minutes

Kit: Pen and journal or any paper

What old, redundant beliefs might be holding you back from expressing yourself and doing what you want to do?

When you have finished, leave space in your journal after this activity, so that you can add any other beliefs that you encounter at a later time.

By the way, it is not to say that parents or significant adults were wrong in giving these messages. In fact, they were just meant to help us through the early years; we were not supposed to carry these 'rules' from childhood through to adulthood.

For some people, these messages from childhood might have been far more damaging and far-reaching than the ones that I have described. It might be tempting to blame those who made the 'rules' for the effect that these beliefs have had on their lives, and feel justified in doing so, but it is a pointless activity. Not only that, it also puts you back into victim mode, leaving you powerless to do anything about it.

Consider just letting it go, forgive them for what they did or didn't do, and move on.

And remember: this forgiveness is something for yourself, you are doing it for you; it is not for the other person. The intention is to give yourself peace, to allow yourself to release the feelings and let go. It does you no good, physically or emotionally, to harbour negative feelings and emotions. Make that forgiveness a gift to yourself, for your own peace of mind and future happiness.

Forgive   Let go   Move on

As an end to the chapter, here are some questions to think about and muse on:

- What do you now believe about the menopause?

- Is it the beginning of a new part of your life or just something to get over?

- Is it a slow slide to the end of your life or a door opening to new possibilities?

- I believe that I can make the most of this time of my life, I may not be able to hold back time, but there are things I can do to help myself. I give in to the process and trust myself and the future.

What do you believe?

Chapter 6

It's a Journey

"Opportunities to find deeper powers within ourselves come when life seems most challenging"

Joseph Campbell

One of the things that helped my thinking the most when I was at the beginning of the menopause was the work of Joseph Campbell and his concept of the Hero's Journey.

The Hero's Journey gave me a way to look at the menopause from the perspective of a story. And every story has a time frame. I also found it useful for thinking and preparing for the kind of things or events that I could expect as I set out on my own intrepid journey.

There is so much more to learn in this fascinating field than I can possibly say here. But in this chapter I'll share with you the overall concept and how it can be useful from the menopause perspective. This time of life is another 'adventure' on your life journey. It is when you learn more about yourself, a time when you can step into a new realm of your own personal power. The concepts here can help you along your journey and add to the understanding you have of the experience and process of your menopause.

The Hero's Journey

I'd like to introduce you to an idea about journeys and heroes, to enable you look at your situation from a different viewpoint. Joseph Campbell researched and wrote about the stories and myths which people from all over the world have told over the centuries and across cultures. He discovered common elements and a pattern in all the stories; he called it 'The Hero's Journey.' There are 12 stages of the journey which I will explain, and afterwards I'll outline what that might mean from the perspective of going through the menopause.

1. Ordinary World – this is the hero's everyday world before the start of the story.

2. The Call to Adventure – the hero is faced with a problem and hears a personal call to do something, like taking on a challenge, going on some sort of adventure.

3. Refusal of the Call – sometimes the hero ignores the call and doesn't take the challenge, perhaps out of fear. Maybe the hero wants to turn back or is not ready to begin

4. Meeting with the Mentor – when the hero decides to take the challenge, there usually appears someone to help. There is the saying 'When the student is ready, the teacher appears'. The mentor helps prepare the hero for the journey, though the journey must be taken alone.

5. Crossing the First Threshold – the hero commits to the adventure, takes on the challenge and steps out of the comfort zone and into the unknown, into a new world. This is the point of no return, you have to go forward.

6. Tests, Allies, Enemies – The Hero discovers personal strengths and weaknesses by being challenged in different ways; and learns how the new world works through friends and foes

7. Approach to the Inmost Cave – this is where the hero faces an enemy, a nemesis. In the myth, it is a dark cave or a very dangerous place.

8. The Supreme Ordeal – the hero has to fight the enemy, facing possible death.

9. Reward – the hero wins the day and gets the prize.

10. The Road Back – the hero prepares to return to the ordinary world.

11. Resurrection –the hero is transformed by the all of these experiences and comes back with a new self-knowledge, insight and understanding.

12. Return with Elixir – the hero returns from the journey with the prize or the treasure and the lessons and uses these to help everyone back in the Ordinary World.

Most people will have experienced this pattern of events several times in their lives. We learn a lot about ourselves and our world during these difficult times. It is through these challenging events that we grow and develop.

On the following pages I have shown a simple example about moving house (in column 2) and then shown how the menopausal journey looks from my perspective (in column 3). It's best to read them a column at a time.

Stage of the Journey	Moving House	The Menopausal Journey
1. Ordinary World	We live in a flat and are quite happy there.	Life is perfectly normal.
2. The Call to Adventure	We decide we would like to have a garden and we need a bit more space.	Quietly at first the symptoms sneak up on me.
3. Refusal of the Call	We did put it off for a little while as the time was not right.	I pay absolutely no attention to the night sweats; I think it is the central heating coming on too early, or the mattress and duvet being too hot.
4. Meeting with the Mentor	In this case, the mentor is the estate agent.	I meet my new friend Ann, who tells me about the menopause from her point of view.
5. Crossing the First Threshold	Find the property, make the decision and put in an offer.	My periods stop and I go to the doctor and decide I will decline HRT and use natural methods to get through it.
6. Tests, Allies, Enemies	Getting the mortgage The solicitor The vendor The planning permission	More symptoms, finding friends who help me and give advice. My homeopathic doctor, Pilates, forgetfulness, hot sweats etc.
7. Approach to the Inmost Cave - the hero faces his enemy	Exchange of contracts and the final signing of the paperwork. Getting answers to all our questions.	I have to come to terms with the fact that I will never have children, that my shape and face have changed and will continue to do so.

8. The Supreme Ordeal - the hero has to fight the enemy, facing possible death	The building of the extension, the new roof and all the unexpected and 'interesting surprises' that we had to deal with. Not to mention the rainy and cold weather for the workmen.	I nearly gave up and let go of myself but I decided to take control, take exercise, change my diet and adjust my lifestyle to accommodate this 'new' body and mind.
9. Reward - the hero wins the day and gets the prize	It's done, the house is in the final stages of completion. The builders leave.	I feel I am doing the best I can, I feel as if I have control and that I have a choice and that my attitude makes all the difference.
10. The Road Back	We prepare to move in.	It's not quite over yet, but I am doing what I can to alleviate my symptoms and work on myself to become the woman I can be.
11. Resurrection - the hero is transformed with a new insight	All the thinking and planning we have done pays off.	I do feel like a different person, I am more at ease with myself, I am happier and I love the person I look at in the mirror.
12. Return with Elixir - the hero returns from the journey	We invite lots of friends round to share our lovely new home, and thoroughly enjoy living in it.	Writing this book allows me to share what I have learned with others.

The example above is based on the stages of the journey as described by Joseph Campbell.

Activity:

Time: at least 30 minutes

On the following page there is an empty grid for you to write in or copy into your journal.

Think back to a time in your life when you were faced with a challenge that you could either accept or ignore – for example: moving house, bereavement, changing jobs, leaving a partner.

What was your journey like? What did you do? Enter your thoughts in the second column.

Then consider your journey through the menopause; fill in the third column.

Stage of the Journey	Example 1	My Menopausal Journey
1. Ordinary World		
2. The Call to Adventure		
3. Refusal of the Call		
4. Meeting with the Mentor		
5. Crossing the First Threshold		

6. Tests, Allies, Enemies		
7. Approach to the Inmost Cave - the hero faces his enemy		
8. The Supreme Ordeal - the hero has to fight the enemy, facing possible death		
9. Reward - the hero wins the day and gets the prize		
10. The Road Back		
11. Resurrection - the hero is transformed with a new insight		
12. Return with Elixir - the hero returns from the journey		

This way of looking at your menopausal journey allows you to think about it more broadly, to see it from a different perspective and to recognise that there may be much to learn and discover along the way. It also gives you a sense of where you are on the path. You can recognise your 'demons and dragons' and see where you need to steel yourself, to dig deep to find your own strength, courage and character from within. Knowing all that, you will emerge wiser and with new insights that would otherwise be invisible to you.

Energies

The hero's journey is also called an archetypal story with archetypal characters; by that I mean the plot that is familiar to all of us, and we know the character types, too. For example, war stories, love stories and tragedies, with warriors, goodies and baddies, lovers, kings and queens.

All of these characters have what we can call 'universal energies'. These are energies we all know and experience at some time or another.

Let's consider just 3 of these Energies: Strength, Compassion, Control. For example, we can look at someone who is worse off than us and experience compassion for them. We can find ourselves in a situation where we are not doing very well and we dig deep for inner strength.

When you think of your journey, and the stage you are at, what sort of energy do you think would be most helpful for you?

Would it be Strength to power you through?

Would it be Compassion, both for yourself and others?

Would it be Control to to help you get order and structure?

Would it be Lightness, Humour and Fun so you could relax and take it less seriously?

If this resonates for you, take some time out to think about it.

Activity

Energy Focus

Time: 20 minutes

- Consider where you are on your physical journey of the menopause, think about what that looks like, feels like and sounds like to you. Then ask yourself which energy would help you to handle it better

- Next, think about the emotional side of the menopausal journey. Which energy would help you with this? Would it be the same energy or perhaps another that I have not mentioned here?

- Write your thoughts and discoveries in your journal

So, in closing this chapter, remember it is a journey and although right now you might not quite be able to see the light at the end of it, you can know that, day by day, you are getting closer to the end than the beginning. There will be good days and not so good days, just keep going and, as you already know, you will be fine.

Chapter 7

Take Time to think

"When we are no longer able to change a situation, we are challenged to change ourselves"

Victor Frankl

It might seem like a luxury, but this change of life is a very important time for you, and it makes sense to devote quality time to thinking about it. Often we just rush through life focusing on the next thing on the to-do-list, sometimes without thinking about where we are going. This menopausal stage is worthy of lots of reflection.

Why? To give yourself time to think, to ponder over how you would like your life to be as you enter this new stage. To give yourself space to muse about how things are currently, how you might change some things to make it better and where you might want to make improvements.

One easy and rewarding way of doing this is to write a journal. You can use it to track your experiences – both good and bad. At times, when we think about the menopause, we tend to focus more on the negatives and forget the positive things. This will help you to get some balance. You will be able to look back over what you wrote and observe how you are changing. You can review what you have written and think about it from a detached perspective, as if you were reading someone else's words. I find it helps me so much as I clarify my thoughts, talk to myself and write about things that I might not want to say out loud to anyone else.

Here is a real excerpt from my own journal to give you a sense of the sort of thing that I write. You might write quite differently, it doesn't matter as long as it helps you to think.

31st January 2006

From my meditation today I learned that I'm more stressed than I thought I was, it was really difficult to switch off. My mind kept racing and going over and over the same things. Company XXX is full of negative energy for me, so do need to let go. I seem to be taking on so much and not getting the recognition for it. "Helloooooo" WAKE UP! You've been going on about this for ages. Let it go! ... It's over and I just need something to replace it with. This is urgent.

Perhaps I can increase my therapy client base by doing some evening therapy sessions and advertise locally and see what comes out of that. Also I could visit the Dr's surgery and see if I can do something there.

I've got lots on my mind, but I need to keep it simple and manageable. I watch myself get so easily distracted and everything becomes more complicated and my thinking gets fuzzy. It's time to make a plan to overcome that.

Wolf medicine is about teaching/writing to share the medicine.

• Shows you how to live a better life

• Tips, techniques, tools

• Talk to you about how to motivate yourself, tell you some secrets

Eagle: conquer the fear and pay attention, reconnect to the element of air, join in the adventure I am co-creating with Spirit. The Universe is giving me the opportunity to soar above the mundane levels of my life. Explore the balance of the spiritual and the earthly.

Now these notes may not mean too much to you, but when I look at them and remember the time I wrote them, there were some revelations within that were most useful, in particular the part about stress and fuzzy thinking.

Note: About the reference to animals Wolf and Eagle: I use cards called 'Medicine Cards' to help me think about things. (Medicine Cards: *The Discovery of Power Through the Ways of Animals* with Hardcover Book by Jamie Sams, David Carson.)

This set of cards comes with a book offering insights and teaching based on the idea that each of the animals has 'medicine' or lessons they can teach us. They were recommended to me by Lydia who starts the day with a meditation on one of the cards.

There are a few ways you can use these beautiful cards, my favourite and most used method is:

1. Shuffle the cards.

2. Shuffle the cards whilst thinking about a problem or a challenge.

3. Lay the cards in an arc or a long line so they are all accessible.

4. Pick a card by running my hand over the spread of cards and choosing the one that seems or feels to be the right one. Sometimes I actually feel my hand tingle when it's over the right card.

5. Look at the card and then read what it says about it in the accompanying book. Each animal has a poem which I write down and think about during the day.

(Note: I have chosen these Medicine Cards, but other people prefer Runes, Angel cards or Tarot cards.)

When I look back over my journal, I see that sometimes I've written page and pages, then at other times just a few bullet points, some pages have little drawings and doodles. None of them are particularly easy to read as I write quite quickly and intuitively.

Your writings are not meant for other people to read, they are for your eyes only. So spelling, grammar and punctuation are not really required.

Another useful function for your journal is when you are not feeling great, you can download all your thoughts about how you feel without overloading friends and family. What you'll find is that just writing about things gets them out of your head and on to paper and that helps you to see things more clearly.

Technique: Visualisation

Everything is created twice, once in our heads when we create the idea, and again in reality where we make it happen and bring it to life.

Visualisation, or visioning, involves thinking of how you want things to be and then, in your imaginary mind, you see yourself acting out that future: seeing what you would see, hearing what you would hear and feeling what you would feel. It is a really powerful process; it's a technique that many highly successful sports people use.

The brain uses the same mental or neural pathways to think about things that have already happened, as well as those that you invent. Basically, our brain can't tell the difference between something that is real and something that is imagined. Therefore, when you visualise a future event, the way you would like it to be, your brain thinks it has already happened. It then uses the vision or the new 'memory' you have designed in your mind as a template for what to create in reality in the future.

You might have seen competitors doing this before a race or an event: standing with their eyes closed, going through the motions of the competition in their mind. I've seen skiers, runners and racing drivers do it. The idea is to visualise yourself in the future, to see yourself doing what you want to do, and feeling how you want to feel. You create an internal mental movie of how you want things to be. Even better, make this is a special multi-sensory movie, add in all the five senses too: what you see, what you hear, what you smell, what you taste and what you feel. The more detail you can put into your movie, the more effective it will be. Think of it as focused day-dreaming. You could see yourself doing your day-to-day activities, being calm and happy. This visualisation creates the road map for your brain to follow, it's like your brain is a computer (which it is) and you are programming what you want from the future. The more you repeat the visualisation, the more powerful the effect. Imagine if you were to do this and repeat it daily ... you will definitely get much more of what you want because you are putting so much attention and focus on it. Every time you run the mental movie in your mind, you reinforce and refine the programme.

There are lots of ways that you can use this technique to help you through the menopause and it is really easy to do, plus you can do it anywhere. Some other examples are:

- You might see yourself calmly dealing with how you feel about hot flushes

- You could picture yourself handling your emotions with your family more effectively; if you have a tendency to get angry, you could see yourself being relaxed and in control

- You could envision yourself in a year's time, at home or at work: happy, relaxed and organised

- You could picture yourself in a meeting that previously you found challenging, being cool, composed and confident

You decide on your time-frame and you decide on the future script that you are going to visualise. Then you just imagine it all as you want it to be.

Why not take a 10 minute break and have a little practice with this.

Activity — visualisation

Time 10 minutes

Think of a situation that you would like to improve, and what your ideal frame of mind would be, and what behaviour or actions will make it better. Then imagine yourself in that situation, create a movie in your head of how the positive version will look. See yourself being on top of things, feeling relaxed and calm and play through the scenario until the happy ending or outcome. You can play it over again to add to it and refine it. The more you repeat that positive internal film, the more likely you are to turn that visualisation into reality.

Note: some people say they find it hard to picture things in their mind. That's OK. It doesn't need to be perfect like a real photograph or a film. For me, I just get a sense of a picture and that works too.

Affirmations

Another way of using this phenomenon is to do affirmations. These are phrases that you repeat to yourself several times a day that can help boost your morale. The classic one is 'Every day in every way I am getting better and better.' The secret is to keep your sentence short and specific, make it positive and in the present tense. Craft it carefully so that it gives you the perfect message for yourself.

You don't actually need to completely believe it in the beginning, but eventually it will become part of your belief system. When I gave up smoking, years ago, I used an affirmation from Dr Allan Carr's book: *The Easy Way to Stop Smoking*. Every time I felt like having a cigarette, I had to say, "I'm a non-smoker and I'm never going to smoke any more". In the beginning, the first few times I said it, it seemed utterly ridiculous that I would be saying those words. However, I persevered with it and now, 19 years later, it is quite true: I am a non-smoker and I'm never going to smoke any more.

Here are some other examples to inspire you as you write your own affirmations. If you need more, there are lots of internet sites offering an affirmation a day, or affirmations for different purposes.

- As I learn to love myself, I find that my life is filled with love and joy

- I am happy with who I am, I love and respect myself and the people around me

- I am comfortable with myself and others

- I am open to the unlimited prosperity of the universe

- I love and approve of myself; I am good enough as I am. I ask for what I want, I speak up for myself, I have power

You'll probably need to work out a way to remind yourself to do it. Some people use post-it notes all around the house, others use symbols. One person I know does it every time they enter the bathroom. It's up to you. The more often you say it, the more you reinforce the belief and the more effective it will be.

Write your own affirmations

Time: 30 minutes

Create your own affirmations to help you overcome negative feelings or thoughts.

Write them on cards or post-it notes. Place them strategically so that you are reminded of them, and say them to yourself several times a day for one month. Use your imagination and be creative with your reminders – put them in your wallet, in the fridge, in your diary, on a mirror you use frequently.

At the end of that month, reflect and write in your journal how your affirmation has helped you.

Role Models

Also create some space in your journal where you can think about role-models. Think particularly of older women whom you respect, who have qualities that you value, skills that you might like to develop, women who inspire you. They can be women from your personal life or famous people. In fact, they might well come from your own network as there seem to be few older role-models who are not either in the media or in politics. Look around you and do a bit of research and see who you can find to inspire you.

Here are just a few examples:

- Barbara Follett: an MP in her 60s – she looks wonderful, speaks very well and lives a full and active life

- Hilary Clinton: US Secretary of State

- Tina Turner: seemingly indefatigable rock star

- Helen Mirren: Actress – gorgeous and still sexy

- Ruby Wax: Comedienne – funny, edgy and energetic

When you are thinking about role-models, it's not necessary to choose just one, you could have several. You can create a kind of composite with the different skills and qualities of the various people rolled into one, if you want.

The main reason for having a role-model is so that you can see in them desirable traits that you can emulate, or perhaps a frame of mind that you can relate to and replicate.

All this is with a view to help you to be more resourceful as you go through the menopause, to help you find different capabilities within to help you handle it. So, on a day when you are feeling a little low, you might ask yourself, 'What would

Margaret Thatcher do now?' or 'What would Joan Rivers say now?'

Of course, your role-models don't necessarily have to be female – if I wanted to lighten up a bit, I might look to Eddie Izzard for inspiration, or I might think of Gandhi if I was looking for calm and strong. If you want to, you can create a page in your journal where you collect names of the people that you admire and look up to, as you find them. The choice is yours.

Future Focus

Some of us are happy with lots of change and find it easy to handle. Others would prefer it if time stood still and things stayed the same, although there are probably things that we are tired of and want to leave behind. As someone once said, 'You can't live your life by looking in the rear-view mirror'. You have to look forward in order to get anywhere.

And if it's true that we won't get our 'old self' back, then perhaps now is the time to start creating your new self, working out how you want to be, how you want your life to be and how you want your world to be.

We can have elements of our old self back BUT we can also reinvent ourselves for this new time of our life, a new incarnation.

So your mission, should you chose to accept it, is to write. Here's what to do...

First, get a book to write in, make sure it is a beautiful one that you really like the look and feel of.

(For example, Paper Blanks have a range of fabulous, luxuriously-bound journals or Moleskine is the legendary notebook that has held the inspirations and ideas of many famous creative people. Or maybe just a simple plain exercise book will be the right thing for you.)

Next, find a lovely pen, pencil or coloured fine-tipped felt pens that you really love to write with.

Place

Then, settle yourself somewhere that will enable you to think in peace. Some people might look for silence, others might prefer more buzz and action. It doesn't necessarily need to be somewhere quiet, just somewhere you can be **undisturbed**. You will know the sort of place you like. Obviously time of year will have some impact on where you choose. Probably not the beach in the middle of winter but, on the other hand, if that suits you, then go for it! You could be at home in a favourite chair, with cushions and a warm throw, or you could go outside.

Some other ideas: a big comfy chair in a hotel lobby, a safe corner in a bookshop coffee shop, a pub or a café, on a bus or a train, a park, some calm green space, by the river – anywhere you like where you can sit comfortably for an hour or so. Be inventive, you never know where your best thinking will happen, so enjoy experimenting.

If you are not really happy being on your own, then practise doing just that a few times. Find somewhere you think looks safe, take a book, get a coffee or tea or soft drink and stay there alone for 30 minutes. Enjoy observing the world going by. Notice the thoughts you have about other people. Pay attention to what you are thinking. You will probably find that no-one really notices you or pays attention to you. Then just take pleasure in being with yourself, claiming your place in the world and doing what you want to do. Some people say that when women get to 40 they become invisible. Well, this is a time when it's a bonus! You can sit on your own and nobody notices. Smiling, I'm saying to you that, unseen, you can think and write to your heart's content.

Time

I recommend you specifically plan some time to do this, and put it in your diary. (You could call it 'A meeting with MySelf'). I can imagine that it would be easy for you to say to yourself, 'Oh, I'll just do that when I'm out and about' or 'I'll just play it by ear'; or you might think that you will do it when you have some spare time. I don't know about you, but I find myself having less and less spare time. It is really easy to get sidetracked by other priorities and tasks, not to mention that tendency that I have been experiencing recently: forgetting what I intended to do in the first place! It is essential that you make and take this time for yourself. Don't leave it to chance; decide that you are going to do it and when, then make it happen.

Questions

So you have decided where and when you are going to think; now here are your questions to ponder, to reflect on and to muse over. There are no right answers and you may answer them differently each and every time you ask yourself the question and that is absolutely fine. Every time you go through the thought processes, you'll refine and clarify your thinking.

Enjoy the thinking and writing and let your thoughts flow where they will. There's no need to censor or evaluate, just let the words come to you. This is just an opportunity for you to catch your thoughts and take time to consider what your current views and ideas are.

1. What have I loved about my life so far?

2. What do I no longer want?

3. What do I want that I don't have?

4.   What would I like more of in the future?

5.   What makes me happy?

There are no right answers, just what is right for you.

Technique: Generative writing

Writing can help us organise our thoughts, come up with new ideas, clarify our thinking or just get stuff out of our heads on to a piece of paper. The mere act of putting pen to paper shifts our thinking into a new realm.

Generative writing is a kind of writing that is very useful when you maybe have a problem, or a challenge, or something is bothering you, or it's just that there is something you want to reflect on. You write about that topic for 10 or 15 minutes, without stopping.

Write

Just write for yourself

Write

Keep writing, don't stop ...

Don't judge, or go back, or cross anything out, just keep writing and see what emerges.

If you do not know what to write, just write what is on your mind, for example something like 'I don't know what to write'. The important thing is to just keep writing and, as you do, your unconscious mind may begin to provide you with solutions. When we run out of words, our subconscious begins to come to the fore. Often this technique gives people new insights into the problem and what they can do about it. I love it because it is an easy process that seems to happen all by itself.

Something to learn: Meditation

So far, I've been suggesting that you do a lot of thinking and writing, now I'm going to suggest that you just STOP, and go inside and think about nothing. I'm suggesting that you meditate. Meditation involves stilling your thoughts and emptying your mind by focusing on a simple object or a sound; if your thoughts start to drift away to something else, you just gently bring yourself back to thinking about the original object.

I love what meditating does for me. I describe it as a 'reset' button for my brain or a drink of water for the soul. It seems to stops the thoughts whirring round in my head; it makes me feel calmer; it helps me to see problems in a different light; it opens up a space where I can be more creative.

When I was at a meditation class, the teacher said this at the beginning, "Breathe in and, just at the moment when you change from the in-breath to the out-breath, there is a short moment of Nothing". Try it now and see for yourself: breathe in and then out and notice that, at the top of the in-breath, there is a moment of stillness and nothing.

That is what meditation allows you to do: have more of those quiet moments of nothing.

It's very easy to learn; you can teach yourself with CDs or tapes, books or you can go to classes. It takes time and practice, but it is so easy and definitely well worth it.

A problem shared

It might be that writing and meditating are just not for you. In that case, you could consider getting together with a group of like-minded women to create a conversation about this time of your life.

- Meeting up to share thoughts and ideas, to support each other, and to chat and talk about the menopause

- Sharing the problem with other people who understand what you are talking about and who may have thought of useful ways of handling things

- Listening about the downsides but, more importantly:

- Encouraging each other to focus on the positives

- Cheering each other up

How to run your group:

1. Decide who you would like to be part of your group. Initially, keep the group numbers small – four or five people; remember, though, that sometimes people won't be able to attend because of other commitments.

2. Identify the reasons for having the group. For example: sharing ideas, coming up with solutions to problems, making people feel better. This is important because you don't want the group to become just a big 'moan about the menopause' session.

3. Make up your 'Rules of Engagement' or 'being together' agreement. The reason for doing this is for everyone to know what is expected of them, to know how to behave and, should you find yourselves being distracted or going off topic, you can easily refer to the agreement to get back on track. Some examples of these rules or guidelines might be:

   a. Everyone gets a chance to speak

   b. No interrupting

    c. No getting on your soapbox

    d. Don't overdo Grumpy Old Woman! Relax and be serene

4. Decide where you are going to meet. Your own home, or take it in turns to host the event, a room in a local pub, a local coffee shop or café?

5. Decide when and for how long. What time of day will be best? What day of the week? For example, would it be midweek in the evening or Saturday afternoon? Two or three hours?

6. Do what you need to do to make sure it happens

7. Finally celebrate and congratulate yourselves on what you have achieved

Action Learning Set (ALS)

One way of making sure your meeting is really effective is to run it like an **action learning set**. This type of approach is often used in business and in situations where people want to learn about something and also to take action as a result of the learning. I was first part of an action learning set when I was doing my Advanced Diploma in Coaching and Mentoring. A group of five of us decided we were going to set up a support group to help us to get through the course, but we wanted more than just support. We wanted an environment where we could learn and develop, where we could challenge and be challenged and we wanted to get maximum value from the time we spent together. The focus is on learning and also taking action as a result of that learning. It's great because it's supportive, interesting and it leads to practical solutions.

The ALS is a disciplined method, where a group of about six people meet regularly, say every month or so, over a period of a year. At the end of that year, they decide if they want to carry on and contract again for another year. This means that group members can bow out gracefully if they want to. As you can imagine, there is an element of commitment to the group and to the process.

There is a clear process to follow at every meeting

You can choose to focus on one person per meeting, or each group member gets a specific time-slot dedicated to them. My preference is for each person who becomes the speaker to have about 20 minutes each.

There are some critical guidelines that everyone must follow. During their 20 minutes, other group members must:

- Listen carefully

- Not interrupt, butt in, offer advice, or be judgmental

- Hear people out and just accept and respect what they hear

- Give no advice unless asked for it

- Not talk about their own situation or tell anecdotes

The 20 minutes gives the speaker the opportunity to talk about their situation, unimpeded and unconstrained. At the end of the time, each group member asks open questions to help the speaker to think differently about their situation, to come up with new ideas and think of different solutions.

A note about **Silence**: Some people feel uncomfortable when there is silence; some hate it and feel they have to say something, that they need to fill the void. In this context, the silence gives us space and time to think. It is during these periods of quiet that we get new ideas and inspiration, we get solutions to problems or new ways of thinking about things. So if the person whose turn it is stops talking, keep quiet while they think of their next thought. Give them that gift of peace where they can reflect in a supportive environment.

Here is how the process works:

1. Each set member reports briefly on what has been happening to them since the last meeting.

2. One at a time, each person in turn has their 20 minutes being the speaker where they describe their situation, problem or challenge.

3. Members of the set ask open questions to help the speaker to think.

4. The set helps the speaker to think about what they will do next and create an action plan.

5. Each set member describes briefly what they have learned and what they plan to do before the next meeting.

6. At the next action learning set meeting, each person reports briefly on what they did differently since the last meeting.

You will need someone to be the facilitator who does the following:

• Establishes the ground rules and keeps everyone on track

• Focuses everyone on the person whose turn it is

• Creates a safe environment for people to explore issues

- Helps the group to identify what they have learned or discovered

This is a wonderful way to spend a few hours, truly listening to others and being listened to yourself. It is a very powerful experience, just to be listened to; this happens so rarely in our everyday lives. Often people are so preoccupied with their own internal or personal world that they only half-concentrate on the people they are with. Nancy Kline in her book *Time to Think* says about listening:

'The quality of your attention determines the quality of other people's thinking.'

Isn't it amazing to think that your listening can have such an effect on someone else's thinking?

It is a very precious gift to both give and receive. Try it and see what you learn from others and, indeed, from yourself.

Chapter 8

Handle the downsides

Throughout this book my message is about helping women to handle the emotional side of the menopause. Encouraging you to think positively, focus on the good things and also to do what you can to make things better. The reality is that the menopause sometimes brings with it some unwelcome side-effects. Our attitude is key to how we deal with this, and there are also practical things we can do.

Here are some that I have experienced and what I have done about it.

Memory

When I was about 15 years old, I remember my mother complaining about her memory being poor: how she would go into a room and forget what she was there for, or she would go to the shop and forget the original thing she was going for and come back with a lot of other things instead. I used to think 'What's the big deal? I forget things, too'. Now I am probably about the age she was then, and I realise that THIS not-remembering is quite different. Back then, I was sure that I would remember what I had forgotten. This time round, I'm not always aware that anything has been forgotten! In some ways it makes life easier, I just do what I remember and then the rest goes away – fantastic! A great reduction in things that stress me out. Of course, the flip-side of that coin is that, later on, I will remember something vitally important that I was supposed to do and didn't. 'Beans on toast for tea again then, darling?'

Here's one example of this symptom that I call 'losing thoughts'. I run a training and development company and I have a very efficient lady called Ann who keeps the books and runs the financial side of the business. Every month I do my expenses and I am very, very careful with receipts so that I can claim back everything I am entitled to. One day she called me and asked where the receipts were for May. I had absolutely NO IDEA! They were not where I usually kept them, nor had I sent them to her. They had completely vanished. This was a month where I had hotel bills and expensive train fares; under normal circumstances, I would have known exactly where that paperwork was, but it had completely disappeared. Fortunately for me, she is of the same age and understands the problem! We muddled through, calling the credit card company to see how much the charges were, contacting the hotel for copies of the bills. Then, about seven weeks later, all these receipts reappeared, in a cupboard that was never a sensible place for them to be. I don't remember putting them in there; I didn't find them when I searched the office from top to bottom; I'm still totally puzzled as to how that happened.

Now I'm learning to write things down to help me to remember, though I often misplace my little notebook of things I don't want to forget. You have to laugh really!

Hot Flushes

What a shock it was when I realised that I was the only person in the room who was much too hot. I struggled to accept that I, too, was going to go through the menopause. Amazingly, up until that moment I had sort of imagined that I would be immune or that it wouldn't happen to me. Duh! In no way had I made a connection in my head between the age I was and the average age at which women become menopausal.

At the time of my very first hot flushes, I was running a training programme with a group of 16 people. I happened to have a kitchen timer with me to keep track of time when they were doing group activities. When I felt one of these flushes start, I turned on the timer. To my surprise and amazement, they only lasted about three minutes. If you had asked me how long they were, I'd have told you about 15 minutes. They seem to go on for such a long time; in fact, for most people they last from three to six minutes. Small fans can be helpful, though fanning yourself with a piece of card can work equally well. You can also try running cold water over your wrists, which brings down the blood temperature.

One friend managed to find a way for me to laugh at the hot flushes. He would tease me gently and show me the funny side of it, often. He made me link them as a reminder about not taking myself too seriously. I now find that I'm usually more amused than anything by that symptom.

As you know, it's important to choose clothes carefully: plenty of natural fibres, lots of layers, perhaps leave out the polo-neck jumpers for a while. For me it's always a dilemma: cotton underwear or something more elegant and sexy! Sarah loves wearing scarves; she told me recently, "These days I can't be bothered with putting them on and taking them off".

Night sweats

It wasn't until my periods stopped that I realised, in fact, it wasn't the central heating coming on too early, or my mattress being too warm, or the duvet being too heavy that was making me feel so hot in bed. Those were actually what we call 'night sweats'. One minute cold and the next minute too hot; throw the duvet off and then put it back on. Repeat at varying intervals. What a nuisance!

Cotton pyjamas have been a godsend. They are not glamorous or sexy but they are absorbent and very comfortable. If you have a few pairs, you can change in the night if you need to and, of course, sleep with the window open!

Tiredness

I don't have quite the same levels of energy that I used to have and I am not able physically to do quite as much as I used to. So now I'm doing my best to avoid overdoing things and I rest a little more. Power naps are also a good idea; this involves breaking away from your activities during the day and taking a nap for about 20 to 30 minutes. The trick is not to allow yourself to get into a complete sleep cycle because, if you do, you might waken feeling drowsy and groggy. A complete sleep cycle lasts about 90 to 100 minutes.

For some people, sleeping can be a problem. Lack of sleep can be brought on by night sweats or being anxious. Often I hear people complain about it, but they don't really DO anything to make it better.

There are obvious things to do, for example: sleep more, go to bed a bit earlier, have long lie-ins at the weekend.

Things to do

1. Create a clean, clear and clutter-free space that is restful and calm.

2. Create a bedtime routine.

3. Lavender on a handkerchief near your pillow.

4. Soothing music.

5. Very comfortable bed linen/nightwear.

6. Create an action plan, or rather in 'inaction plan' of what to do when you wake in the night and things start to go around in your head.

Your 'inaction plan' might involve counting sheep or a relaxation technique, just don't automatically let your brain wake up and start whirring around! When I went through a phase of not sleeping well because of a house move, I used to keep a pen and a big notebook at the side of the bed. If I woke up, I would keep my eyes closed, write down the thoughts that were beginning to wake me and promise myself that I would attend to them in the morning. That way, I didn't lose the thought but I didn't lose any sleep over it either.

There are some wonderful audio CDs available which provide music and sounds that get your brain working at the speed you need for particular activities.

Simply put, our brainwaves operate at four different rates which are:

Beta Waves: our normal waking state where we are alert and working.

Alpha Waves: when you are relaxed and creative energy starts to flow.

Theta Waves: where brain activity slows almost to the point of sleep; often inspiration happens at this stage, you get flashes of imagery and you can also get a sense of floating. It is also known as the 'twilight state'; Einstein was in this state when he had his 'Eureka' moment about the speed of light where he imagined he was riding on a sunbeam.

Delta Waves: which is during deep, dreamless sleep. If you are waking in the middle of the night and your brain starts racing, then it will be harder for you to go back to sleep. You might want to try audio CDs that are designed to encourage that Delta Wave brain activity.

Websites to try: www.brainsync.com and www.pzizz.com

Body changes

Our bodies do change as we get older, that is a fact. What we can do is to make the most of them, take great care of them and keep them in peak condition. Some people treat their car with more care than they treat their body. A service here and, when the time comes, an MOT there. It's worth considering this: you can replace your car and even go and buy a brand new one; we know that you can't get a new body, not really. The question is: How can we keep this body we have in tip-top condition because it has to last us for another thirty years or more?

Various advertisements promise the 'elixir of youth' and show us pictures of models whose photographs have been digitally enhanced. Healthy eating, exercise, drinking plenty of water and getting plenty of sleep will probably do more for us than expensive creams and lotions. I'm not saying give up the creams and lotions, what I'm saying is look after the inside as well as the outside.

What about in the bedroom?

Oh, how I have agonised over whether to mention sex or not. In fact, that's part of the problem, isn't it? We don't talk about it. Many of us keep this to ourselves, perhaps because it's not so easy to talk about, and also we might not have the right language readily available to describe what and how we feel.

The emotional side of this involves loss of libido; some women say they just don't feel like it, that sex is not as exciting, stimulating or rewarding as it once was. This can be a vicious circle: it's not so enjoyable so we want it less, then it's not that great and it becomes even less appealing. All this leads to a general loss of interest.

Other factors which come into play are that some women feel less attractive, and are more self-conscious of their body. I know that if I have put on a few pounds and have not been doing regular exercise, first of all I feel less flexible and also I'm just not as physically able to do it. I have found that a few weeks of going to the gym or exercise classes and a sensible eating plan really make a big difference to my confidence and enthusiasm. Some women say they feel too tired, others say they are just not turned on in the same way they once were.

Carol said, "I haven't had sex for about seven years, there just doesn't seem to be time, and I'm not really bothered or interested. I find the idea of it daunting. I miss the closeness and the intimacy, but it just seems to be gone from my life. Terry and I, we don't talk about that sort of thing, I've no idea how I'd even start to bring up the subject."

The physical side is also changing; vaginal atrophy is one of the symptoms, which means that it can become tighter and more painful. Remember, the vagina is like a muscle: use it or lose it. Dryness can also be a problem, though there are water-based lubricants or creams that you can get on prescription from your doctor. Janice swears by vitamin E capsules, she pierces them with a pin and applies it to the area, both inside and out.

Here are some things you can do:

- Talk to your husband or partner about it, so that they can understand

- Make sure your bedroom helps you feel relaxed and the lighting is low and soft

- Reduce your expectations of yourself, don't judge, be kind to yourself

- You might consider revving up your fantasies; after all, in your head you can be who and what you want to be

- Try some sexy lingerie, something that covers and reveals at the same time

- See your doctor, perhaps an oestrogen cream might help

- Do your pelvic floor exercises to keep those muscles in tip-top condition. You can feel your pelvic floor muscles if you try to stop the flow of urine when you go to the toilet, though don't use that as the exercise. To strengthen these muscles, sit comfortably and squeeze and release them 10-15 times in a row. Avoid holding your breath, or tightening your stomach, buttock, or thigh muscles at the same time. It will take a bit of time before you start to notice the results, but you should notice an increase in the sensitivity you experience during sex. It also helps with the inadvertent leak when laughing, coughing or running. You should carry on doing the exercises, even when you notice them starting to work.

If you do want to improve your sex life, you'll need to give it some attention, some thought and some time.

Whilst I am not a medical expert, and this book is not so much about the physical side of things, nevertheless the mind and body are connected so here are some things that have worked for me.

Drinking enough water?

Doctors recommend that we should drink six to eight glasses of water a day to keep ourselves well-hydrated; this is vital for us, both physically and mentally. Recent reports have stated that we need to drink two litres a day, but that has been disputed as some of our water intake comes from our food. Generally, we lose between one and two litres of water a day, which we need to replenish, not only from what we drink but also from what we eat. Also, at this time of life, we will also be losing more water through hot flushes and night sweats, so we need to make sure that we keep well-watered. Research has shown that a 2% drop in hydration can cause a 20% drop in performance and lead to tiredness and lethargy. I find the two litres works for me, I always feel better if I drink that amount of water per day. I suggest that you track your own water intake and energy and see whether making adjustments will improve how you feel.

Eating healthy food

This is a really obvious one; when I pay little attention to what is good for me to eat, I don't feel good. Sometimes I've got this blind spot where I'll choose something that is convenient but not necessarily good for me, without even thinking about how I might feel afterwards. I'm probably not the only person to long for a big slice of toast or piece of cake, knowing that it will make me feel sluggish, sleepy and bloated. I'll scoff it, enjoy it in the moment and, barely 10 seconds afterwards, be filled with regret. It's a lesson I am still learning! When I eat well I feel much better. Fresh vegetables and fruit, protein, and just a little carbohydrate works for me. Each and every body is different, so different things will work for different people. The trick is to experiment with what works for you. Get honest about what you are eating. Do you have good intentions, but find yourself eating junk to save time or for convenience? Do you find you crave foods that you know are not really nourishing for you?

Do you skip meals or forget to eat? Are you always 'on a diet'? Do you eat for comfort? Give this some time and some thought so that you are consciously aware of your eating habits.

One great way of doing this is to keep a food diary. All you need is a small notebook that is easy to carry with you. Make a note of *everything* you eat and drink, and pay attention to how you feel afterwards. Does what you have eaten energise and nourish you or does it make you feel tired? When I did this, I discovered that if I ate a bacon sandwich I would be asleep an hour later!

Exercise

Again, this is another obvious one. It is vital to keep active and take exercise. I find that when I exercise the hot flushes are reduced. In an ideal world, we should do some form of cardio-vascular activity four times a week for at least 30 minutes I'm told, plus some weight-bearing exercise to help our bone strength. Get your body moving. Yoga is particularly good as it helps both body and mind.

Stop for a moment and be honest with yourself about how much exercise you take. Is it really enough? If not, what could you easily add to your daily routine that would improve this?

Some other things to try:

Cutting out wheat: this may be an old wives' tale, but I find the less wheat I eat, the fewer hot flushes I get. It's definitely worth a try. Try it for about a week and see if it makes a difference for you.

Herbs: black cohosh, red clover, agnus castus and sage can help. There are many herbal remedies on the market that can alleviate hot flushes and night sweats. Tessa recommends **Meno-herbs,** saying, "I started taking these and the hot flushes stopped almost immediately, it's brilliant". Olga suggested **Menopace**, saying, "I took these and really didn't notice any symptoms". Having no medical training, I won't recommend anything other than to suggest you try things out for yourself.

Heather Fairbairn runs an organisation called Menopause Support, helping women prepare for and cope with the menopause; she says "Changing your diet and including carefully selected supplements certainly help many women through the menopause. Some women find alcohol, coffee and hot spicy foods bring on hot flushes but eating foods rich in phytoestrogens (such as beans and seeds) and including good quality Vitamin E and C supplements can reduce their frequency and intensity considerably."

Snacks: check out what you typically tend to snack on, decide whether that is good for you or not. I used to have a cup of tea and a biscuit. Even though the biscuits were made of oats, they still contained sugar, so I got the sugar rush and then the subsequent come-down. I now go for fruit, nuts and seeds which seems to work well for me.

With all of the downsides I have mentioned, the secret is to recognise them and do everything you can to improve the situation. Acknowledge what you are thinking and feeling. Give yourself time to reflect on it, and then do something about it; take action. Whenever you hear yourself complaining about the menopause, follow those thoughts with a positive idea and make this a habit. If you do this, you will begin to change your attitude which, in turn, will change how you feel about the menopause and that will make it easier to handle it.

Reduce your focus on the negative, concentrate on what you want and then do what you can to help yourself to get there.

Finally, to wrap up this chapter, ask yourself the following questions and write the answers in the box below:

What are the three things that I am going to do something about as a result of reading this chapter?

1.

2.

3.

What will be the benefits? To me? To the people around me?

How might I sabotage myself, and what shall I do to prevent that?

What simple actions am I going to take and when?

Note: This does not necessarily mean that you need to find huge life-changing actions to take; just a few little changes will make all the difference.

Chapter 9

Being Self-Confident

Confidence is a firm belief in one's powers, abilities, or capacities.

"You gain strength, courage and confidence by every experience in which you really stop to look fear in the face"

Eleanor Roosevelt

Confidence. The word has its roots in Latin and it simply means having faith in yourself. It is about having self-belief and self-esteem, and also trusting that you are enough. I think that menopause symptoms can easily derail our confidence. Feeling hot and bothered, losing words and fuzzy thinking can all get in the way of feeling self-assured. So in this chapter you will find some techniques and resources to help you boost your belief in yourself.

An interesting way of thinking about confidence is that it might seem like a state of mind, but it is also requires taking action. Here's what I mean by this: some years ago, on a skiing holiday, I went to ski school in the mornings because I wanted to improve. I was not a very confident skier; I was a bit frightened, not only of the heights, but also the speed, on some days the combination of both was terrifying! Ski slopes are categorised by colour: green being the easiest, blue is less easy, increasing in difficulty to red and then black for the most challenging. On confident days, I skied reasonably well; I could get down a red run fairly easily and enjoy it. On the days when I doubted myself, the same runs would seem impossible to get down. I would stand at the top, looking down at the steep expanse of white, stiff with fear and my mind in a panic knowing that the only way down the mountain was to either ski or walk. And let me tell you, walking down (carrying the skis) was not, in any way, a sensible option.

One day the instructor said, "To start, you must LEAN down the mountain", meaning you have to shift your entire body-weight forward and lean towards the tips of your skis, facing down the slope, essentially **launching** yourself on to the piste. This gives you momentum and speed, makes the skis run more smoothly and also makes it easier to turn. (You have to be able to turn, otherwise it's straight down the middle at about 90 miles an hour – bad idea!)

What a dilemma and a paradox: paralysed by fear one goes nowhere; to get somewhere you have to throw yourself down the mountain.

Although you may not have been skiing, or shared my experience, I'm sure you can think of situations that you have been in where you have had similar feelings and worked out that you just had to have faith, jump in and hope for the best. As I think back, here are some of the things that spring to mind for me:

Learning to skip where two girls turn the rope and you have to run in and jump with it. Terrifying: What if I get it wrong? What if they get annoyed with me for messing up?

First time in the driving seat: Oh my, what if I can't stop? What if I hit something? What if I have to buy my Dad a new car because I've crashed this one?

Jumping down the escape slide of a jumbo jet, practising for an emergency: Crikey, it's really high! I'm scared of heights, I can't do this! Swiftly followed by: If I don't do this, there goes my career at British Airways! – just go for it – and then squealed all the way to the bottom. What a hoot when I look back at it!

It might be useful to stop now and think about these events for a few moments and consider what you learned from them.

Activity – learning from my own experiences

Time: 15 - 20 minutes

Kit: Journal and pen

Settle down in a comfy place, ready to reminisce.

Think back to at least one situation where you overcame either your self-doubt or your fear. Make a note in your journal, and write down what you learned from those experiences. (Notice if what was once very serious indeed can now be viewed as amusing.)

Take five minutes or so to pause and think about what you learned at the time.

Jot down at least three learnings or lessons that you got from the experience.

Ask yourself 'What else did I learn that I didn't notice then but I do now?'

The decisions we take at those times are testimony to our ability to be confident, to trust in ourselves and to do what needs to be done. There are five key elements that always seem to be present in any situation where we need confidence; here they are:

The five keys to confidence

- Knowing what you want

- Self-awareness: knowing yourself and understanding why you do what you do

- Taking Control

- Believing in yourself, trusting your ability to get there

- Doing what you need to get the result you want

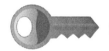 ### 1. Knowing what you want

Often when I ask coaching clients what they want, they start by giving me a long list of what they **don't** want. We seem to find it easier to think of unwanted things. The problem is this: using what we don't want as a goal to work towards is useless. Imagine this: a fairy godmother appears ands says benevolently with a beautiful smile, "You can have one single wish, any wish you want. What's it going to be?" I'm thinking that you would make sure you answered carefully and said exactly what you had in mind – or would you? There might be someone out there who'd say, "I wish I knew what I wanted, I can't make up my mind!"

Anyway, the point is to work out exactly what you want and where you want to get to. You can use the old familiar Mnemonic SMART to help you get clear on your outcome.

Specific

When you think of your goal, what exactly do you want?

Poor example:	I want to write a book.
Better example:	I want to write a book that will help women deal with the emotional side of the menopause.
Even better example:	I want to write a book that will help women deal with the emotional side of the menopause, which is practical, light-hearted and easy to read.

The more specific and clear you are on the description of your outcome, the easier it will be for you to work out what to do to achieve it.

Measurable

'What gets measured gets done'. This is an old adage but it stands the test of time.

If you can measure the results, it makes it really easy for you to track how you are doing, to know where you are and to check if you have reached your goal.

For example, I can measure how many chapters and pages I have written.

Achievable

Make sure that the goal does not overstretch you.

Writing a book in a week = not achievable

Writing the first draft of a book in three months with the help of a coach = achievable

Realistic

Check that your goal is realistic to make sure you set yourself up for success based on your physical capabilities and your surroundings.

Be careful on this one though. There is a successful basketball player in the American major league who is 5ft5 when the average is about 6ft7. At the outset, his goal of playing in the top flight of US basketball might have seemed somewhat unrealistic. Whilst other people might not believe that we can achieve what we set out to do, if you think it is realistic, then, by all means: You Go For It!

Timed

Make sure you have a completion time and date and year for your goal. 'The end of February' is not enough.

Every year has an end of February – We could postpone to 2011, 2015, 2019 ...

What if my subconscious made the date the 29th February – I'd have to wait till the next Leap Year!

I once had a coaching client who decided she wanted a new job; she chose her completion date as Anzac day. Three days before that date, she called to tell me about her new job! It is amazing how your focus and motivation can change when you specify a date. (If you want to be even more precise, you can add the time of day, too!)

Five years ago, I decided I was going to write a book; I could have been more specific about the time, but here I am, typing like a woman possessed.

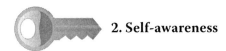 **2. Self-awareness**

This is about knowing and accepting yourself, understanding why you do what you do. For many women, one of the benefits of the menopause is that they have come to a time of their life when they are no longer so worried about what other people think of them. They are more accepting of themselves, both how they look and how they feel.

Some women feel as if they are out of control, at the mercy of their symptoms and feelings. This is especially true for women who feel that they are defined by the people around them, for example their husbands, families or partners. Some women find it hard to think about themselves as an individual in their own right, some feel that how other people describe them, or see them, is how they are. This is not the only truth; you are definitely more than just that. If this is you, make sure you take some time to think about your strengths and qualities, the things that make you uniquely you.

Self-awareness and self-acceptance go hand-in-hand. This key will help you to unlock more of who you are.

On the one hand, you might say it's time to accept who you are, and recognise that this is the best it can get but, on the other hand, who knows what you still have to learn about yourself? You are so much more than you think you are. You have capabilities and qualities that you are still to discover. Revel in this new incarnation of you that is unfolding. Look to the positive and find an even more confident version of yourself.

Some people feel that this time of life is the end of 'themselves'. Well, in some respects that might be true, but there is still so much more to find out and you might like to think of it this way:

You are perfectly fine as you are – there is no-one else as good, at being you, as you are.

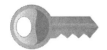 ### 3. Taking Control

Taking control of your own life is key to building your confidence, so is taking responsibility for what happens to you. For as long as we look for other people to blame and make excuses for ourselves, we put ourselves in a powerless situation. If you stop making excuses and blaming other people, then you are able to make a decision, do something about the situation and move on.

> *Sandra believed that she could not get a promotion because her boss was about to retire; he was not much interested in his job or bothered about developing his team any more. She didn't bother to talk to anyone about her aspirations for the future because she thought it was pointless. She wasn't really doing her best work either, as she thought that no-one really cared. When I asked her what she could do to take control for herself, she came up with several ideas which included: being brave and asking the boss about it, talking to the HR department about other opportunities and developing her network of colleagues so that she knew of any up-and-coming vacancies. She also started being more conscientious, and took on a project where she was able to learn new skills and also to meet other colleagues. This change of attitude was noticed by everyone and she was soon happily installed in a new department with a new boss who really values what she does.*

By the way, most people have many areas of their lives which run well and where they are in control and make things happen the way they would want. Then, occasionally, something goes out of balance or changes and the person finds themself making excuses, blaming the situation or other people. Often I get called in as a coach when someone has got stuck in their reasons and their excuses and can't find a way out – usually they just don't recognise that they can do something about it.

Here's another way of looking at this:

Imagine a situation where you are not very confident. On the one hand (at the left side of the line) you can give reasons, make excuses and justify why you are not able to do anything about it. Perhaps you are making it someone else's fault. On the other hand (at the right side of the line) you could take responsibility to do what you can, take control of the situation and take action.

At one end of this line are the times when you make excuses; at the other are the times when you decide what you want and what you need to do to make that happen.

Excuses ←————————————————→ **Control**

At this end of the line are the people who say things like:	At this end of the line are the people who say things like:
It's not my fault I can't help it It's their fault, they made me do it	I'll do what I can It's up to me to do something about it I can change this

I can understand that you might not want to see yourself as someone who acts as if they are at the Excuses end of this line. If you are the type of person who always tries to blame someone else, or find reasons as to why it's not you, or you look for excuses, then that might be where you are. Here's the problem with this: for as long as you are arguing for it not being your fault, at the same time you are effectively saying to yourself, 'I can't help it, there's nothing I can do', which then means that you are powerless. For as long as you are upholding the excuses and justifying them, you are stuck and not able to take control and move forward. Here's an example of mine:

Excuses ◄─────────────────────────► **Control**

I want to lose weight • It's hard to find time to go to the gym because I am so busy • I'm away from home often staying in hotels and I can't easily get the right food to eat • Losing weight is just so much harder when you get older.	• I've heard my own excuses, but I'm going to do something about this • I'm going to make it a long- term plan to make sure I do some exercise three times a week • I'm going to reduce my portion sizes by a quarter

If I continue to justify the stuff in the box on the left, I'm just not going to get the result that I want, so:

Stop making excuses and blaming other people, take control and ask yourself this:

What is the smallest step that I can take to move the situation forward?

Whatever the answer is that you give: Do It!

Do you 'get in the way of yourself'? Do you stop yourself from doing things you want to do? Some of us will sabotage ourselves. Most of us will have Avoidance Strategies. These are things that we distract ourselves with when there is something difficult or important that we want to avoid doing. Sometimes we do this consciously, but more often than not it is an unconscious thing. For example, if I have a difficult telephone call to make to the bank and I find myself 'just cleaning out the fridge first,' or I've got expenses to do, but I can find any number of other activities to do instead which, by the way, are less important. You will know which things you seek to avoid.

Identify your Avoidance Strategies and when you realise that is what you are doing, get yourself back on track. Focus on what you really should be doing; break the task down into bite-size chunks and Just Do It.

Also, at this point stop to consider if you are avoiding something so successfully that you are *never* going to do it. For me it was learning Spanish. When I was 18, I decided that it was an ability that I wanted, it was on my list of 'things to do' for years, but I never did it. It just wasn't important enough. Eventually, I finally gave up on it and I've never regretted it. So: Make a decision: either do it or don't – but don't whinge on about it! Give yourself a break and just let it go!

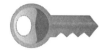 **4. Believing in yourself, trusting your ability to get there**

In our lives we have all faced challenges that we have got over, and there will be more to come, and we will get over these, too. We know that people can handle the most extraordinary events and come through the other side. As time passes, we can forget about those really hard lessons we have had in life, or the huge efforts we have made to overcome problems. Each and every one of us will have had huge difficulties that we have dealt with and put behind us. It's easy to forget the strengths and qualities that got us through those times, but they are there within us as our internal resources.

When it comes to being confident, the first step is to trust yourself and then to do the best you can. As you think about difficult situations where you would like more confidence:

- Think back and see if it is similar to any previous events, so that you can draw on your own experience

- Ask yourself what qualities, skills and inner resources you have that you can draw on in this situation

- Do you know anyone else who has dealt with this; what did they do?

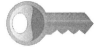 ## 5. Doing what you need to get the result you want

Take action! You know how much energy goes into putting things off and waiting and worrying. Work out what you need to do and organise it into manageable chunks so you are not trying to do too much all at once.

Stop procrastinating! Putting it off until tomorrow doesn't help, it just postpones the inevitable. Focus your attention on how pleased you will be with yourself when it is done.

Something that is a challenge on a Monday morning will not be any easier by Thursday. In fact, it will feel more difficult, plus you will have expended untold energy NOT doing it. Instead of the dread of doing the thing, look forward to being pleased with yourself. Usually, most things are never as hard as we imagine they are going to be.

Just start – that is the secret.

What do you say to yourself?

Earlier in this chapter I talked about the fact that you are fine – in fact You are perfect as you are. You are unique and precious and special. There is no-one else like you, and you are the best You there is!

If, you are not entirely convinced that you are perfect as you are, notice what you were saying to yourself. We can be our own worst enemy: criticising ourselves, berating ourselves for inadequate performance, doubting our abilities, questioning our decisions. At this time of life, it is really easy to look at ourselves and find ourselves wanting. I'd like you to stop doing that now and be your own inner coach/ cheerleader/ motivation guru/ best friend.

We all have an inner voice, an internal dialogue that goes on inside our head. It often comments on what is going on in the world around us, making judgements on other people and ourselves. For some people, it is a critical little voice that says things like, 'You shouldn't have done that', 'What will they think?', 'You're not good enough for this'. The purpose of that inner dialogue is to keep us safe, to stop us from making an idiot of ourselves and to help us to do a good job. Sometimes it is not helpful. Have you noticed also that it has a particular tone of voice?

Fortunately, what you may not know yet is that we do actually have control of this inner dialogue. *You* are in charge of that voice and how it sounds.

Here's a quick experiment: think of what you say to yourself when you have done something really stupid or silly. (For me it is a very sarcastic and nasty 'Urgh, what an idiot' or 'Well done, that was really clever', but said in a really critical, nasty and cutting tone.) Now say that same thing to yourself, but change the voice to the tone you would use when talking to a baby, or your own very sexy-tone voice – deep, soft and whispery; or, alternatively, Minnie Mouse's voice. Play around with this sentence in your head, using different tones of voice and notice that the harsh words don't have the same impact when they are said in a different tone.

So if you hear yourself using that negative manner and tone:

1) Ask yourself what would be a more positive message that you could replace it with.

2) Decide on a more helpful tone of voice.

3) Consider if you were your own best friend, helping you in the situation, what would you say to yourself?

Then, all you do is change that internal dialogue and the tone of voice.

Perfection and the 80/20 rule

Are you always looking for perfection? This can completely wear you out. Perfection is an illusion, it is like an oasis in the desert calling you to it but, when you approach it, it vanishes. It takes up lots of time and you can end up striving for something that is irrelevant. Some people are never satisfied with what they achieve. If you have a strong need to be perfect, this can take up a lot of your energy; it's time-consuming and you may always find yourself being disappointed by your failure to achieve it.

You have probably heard of Pareto's Law, also known as the 80/20 rule. It was originally a theory on the distribution of income: i.e. 20% of the population earns 80% of the income.

It applies in other areas, too. For example:

- If we have a task to do that we want to avoid, we will often spend 80% of the time on the avoidance activities and then 20% of the time actually doing the task. My Income Tax would be a good example: I spend weeks putting it off and then, once I get round to it, it's done in no time

- Thinking about clothes in your wardrobe, you probably wear 20% of your clothes 80% of the time

- Perhaps you spend 80% of your time thinking of other people and doing things for them, and 20% on yourself

I'm not suggesting that you stop things before they are complete, or don't do the detail and finishing touches. What I am proposing is that, when you feel the need to complete something to perfection, stop and think to yourself: have I done enough? Can I stop now? Think of the 80/20 rule. Will the extra effort I put in here actually deliver perfection and is it worth the time and effort to achieve that? One sentence that I find useful when I am in perfection mode is 'Good enough is good enough'.

Isabelle is a full-time carer for her husband. They are very sociable people, they love having friends round to the house. She is a great cook and, in the past, she always made breakfast, lunch, afternoon tea, and/or dinner for her guests – depending on how long they were staying. She is realising now that she just does not have the time to make it perfect like she used to. If you think of the 80/20 rule, she would put 80% of her effort into the 20% of the visit time that would be spent on eating.

When I suggested that she did the opposite of what she usually did and reduce the catering to a bare minimum, initially she was not enthusiastic about the idea. However, she gave it a go. Now, if you stay overnight, she announces that breakfast is self-service and everyone is happy to serve themselves. Sometimes you get to make your own sandwiches too!

Now they still have lots of visitors, but she is less stressed and pushed for time and she has more energy. She realises that the most important thing is the company, not the catering.

So if you want to free up some time, reduce stress and get more control, then take some time to think about the 80/20 rule and see where it could help you change some areas of your life.

Assertiveness

This is key to being confident. Assertiveness is standing up for yourself and what you believe in, asking for what you want. Occasionally people mistake assertiveness for aggressiveness, especially if someone has previously been very passive and is now saying what they think. The trick is to aim for a win-win situation. There is a simple three-step structure to help you to work out how to say what you want:

1. Listen, and show you understand

2. Say what you think or feel

3. State what you want to happen

When you want to make your point, it is easiest if you can get to the point quickly. This three-step approach helps you to do that.

Remember: Keep calm, avoid being judgemental (the other person did what they did, without thinking of you or considering the impact it may have had on you). Accept that they have a different viewpoint; that is quite normal and acceptable.

Being Assertive – saying it ...

1. Listen, show you understand

See the other person's point of view. Empathise; put yourself in their shoes. Hear them out. Make sure you have fully thought through what their position might be and what they might need from the situation. Remember you are aiming for win-win.

Explain the situation as you see it, calmly and objectively, and keep to the point; don't drag in any other awful things they've done; keep it short.

Don't theorise; stick to describing what's happening, not *why* you think it's happening.

A useful way of starting is to say, for example:

"I can see you are busy at the moment ..."

"I appreciate that you must be tired ..."

"I realise that ..."

Avoid the word 'but'. For example, you might usually say, "I can see you are busy at the moment but we need to discuss plans for the weekend".

There is a phrase that says, "Everything before 'but' is b******t" – the 'but' negates everything that has been said at the beginning of the sentence and it can put people on the defensive. Use 'and' instead.

For example, "I can see you are busy at the moment *and* we need to discuss plans for the weekend".

It feels really weird the first time you say it like this, but it is brilliant for avoiding confrontation. Some people say they can't say it because it is not grammatically correct. What you will find is that the other person doesn't really notice and they don't feel as if they have been rebuffed. (Try it next time you are in disagreement: replace the BUT with AND then see what happens – it's wonderful).

2. Say what you think or feel

You can be honest, no-one can argue with how you feel. Use just one or two words to describe the feeling:

I feel annoyed ...

I feel disappointed ...

I feel irritated ...

I feel disheartened ...

Acknowledge **your** feelings, own them as your responsibility. 'I'm cross' not 'You're making me cross.'

Acknowledge **their** feelings. Empathise by putting yourself in the other person's shoes. It makes it easier for them, they realise that you have considered their point of view and they don't have to make an effort to make you see their point of view.

Note: 'I feel you should put the lid back on the toothpaste' is **not** a feeling! It is a statement dressed up as a feeling.

3. State what you want to happen

Be open, positive and straightforward without insistence or apology. Explain exactly what you need to happen so the situation can be resolved. Be realistic and also prepared to compromise.

Ask assertively; don't demand or manipulate. Respect the other person; this will help your self-respect.

Use 'I' as in 'I want you to ...'

Outline what will happen:

- If the other person does what you want. For example, you
  will be happier, or you will less irritable, or you will work
  harder

- If they don't do what you want; outline the negative effects
  or punishment (don't make empty threats)

It's up to you to decided whether you prefer to use the positive
or negative consequences to finish on. It will depend on the
situation.

And finally ... keep to the point, be calm; you want a win-win
situation for both parties.

Here's how it all comes together: three easy sentences with no
waffle or going round the houses.

"I realise that you have planted these trees to give you privacy
in your garden.

I feel frustrated and annoyed, because they block out the sun
on my patio in the afternoon.

I would like you to reduce the height of them by two feet.

That way we can both have what we want – you still have your
privacy and I get the sunshine."

Qualities and Strengths

You have unique qualities, no-one else on the planet has the same combination of strengths, skills, knowledge and experience that you have.

Here's the funny thing though: there are things that we are exceptionally good at, that we find really easy and we often assume that because we find these things so easy:

a)   Everyone else can do it

b)   If it's so easy then it can't be so special

c)   We don't even notice the special skill in the first place

Years ago, I ran a training course that was designed for 12 participants – six of them came from the IT (Information Technology) section of the company, and six of them were from the airline cabin crew community. When we spoke to them about strengths and qualities, we found that the IT team did not value their attention to detail and their ability to analyse and manipulate data. The cabin crew did not value their ability to keep calm and smile under pressure and to handle the demands of the travelling public. Neither group saw their particular skills as special and assumed that everyone could do what they did.

An activity to help you to recognise your strengths:

Get a sheet of A4 paper, divide it into four boxes and label each box as shown below. Keep the sheet of paper handy and make a note every time you come across something you are good at doing, or not, and something you like doing, or not. Keep noting items in the four areas for a few days, then stop when the boxes are full. Take a look at the things you like doing and the things you are good at and ask yourself 'What qualities might this activity suggest that I have?'

Make a note of the quality in a different colour pen. You might find that some demonstrate more than one quality.

This is not the time to be shy or coy, or even modest. It is for your eyes only, so be brave and honest – no-one will censor or disagree. Really look for the quality that is implicit. For example, 'I really love doing jigsaw puzzles'. Qualities from that might be patience and an eye for detail.

If this is not coming naturally to you, try asking other people, friends, family or colleagues what they think you are good at.

You may be pleasantly surprised by what they say.

I like doing	I'm good at
I don't like doing	I'm not good at

If you are interested in doing some more on this, here is a wonderful book about it.

Now, Discover Your Strengths: How to Develop Your Talents and Those of the People You Manage by Marcus Buckingham and Donald O. Clifton. There is an access code inside the back cover which allows you to do an online questionnaire to discover your own strengths and talents. It's really useful and interesting.

(Tip: don't buy a second-hand copy as the access code may have been used already by the previous owner.)

Body language

Our confidence shows in our body language, our posture reflects the way we feel and, at the same time, the way we feel shows in our posture. Think about how you usually stand and walk. Do you give off a confident vibe? Do you stand tall and straight? Do you walk in a purposeful way?

When you walk into a room do you stride, glide or slide in so no-one notices?

When a person is depressed, you can see it in their body language. Often their head will be bowed, they will look down frequently and their shoulders might look as if they bear the weight of the world.

Experiment: playing with body language

Here's something to try.

Part 1

Imagine for a minute that you are bored, tired and fed-up. Now sit in a chair, exactly the way you would sit if you were bored, tired and fed-up. You might have to sigh a lot, droop your shoulders, drop your head, let your facial muscles fall, huff and puff as if you were bored stiff. Notice as you do this that, by changing your body position, your body language begins to affect how you feel. And even though you started off just pretending that you were bored, tired and fed-up, you may well actually be feeling bored, tired and fed-up, too! So, move on quickly to the next part.

Part 2

Now imagine yourself to be totally motivated! Fully energised! Absolutely brimming with oomph and 'get up and go'! Go on! Do it now! Really exaggerate and turn up the intensity! At the same time, change your posture and body language to match that mode. Perhaps your shoulders go down and back, you might smile, or feel your face lift, your spine straighten. You might breathe in quickly to oxygenate yourself ready for action. You might want to put the book down for a couple of minutes while you do this and really get into how it feels.

You will probably notice that, even though you started off by just imagining, or pretending you were really energised, actually you have started feeling that way.

What this activity is intended to demonstrate is that our body language affects how we feel. So, if you are not feeling the way you want to feel, change your body position, your head, shoulders and breathing, try standing tall and straight, breathing in and out slowly, from the bottom of your diaphragm. What you'll find is when you 'put on' different body language, you feel and act differently.

Act as If

As someone once said to me, "Just pretend: 'Act As If' and you will be fine".

I was pleased that I had learned that before I had my first real hot flush; here's why.

I was a trainer in a room with about 18 people, running a four-day Influencing Skills course, talking about being open and honest, when all of a sudden I felt a heat emanating from below and behind my ears. It was different from any sensation I had felt before, so I knew it was something new. At the same time though, it felt like the feeling you get when you are embarrassed. That heat and feeling took me straight back to childhood – not to any specific moment, but to a familiar feeling of self-consciousness, discomfort and embarrassment that I would get when I had done something wrong. Even though I knew there was no reason to feel that way, at that moment, the physical sensation of rising heat brought back those old familiar feelings. I was acutely aware of how I felt, I assumed that the group could see that I had changed colour to a mild shade of scarlet, and I started to worry that the audience would think I was lying about what I was saying. What a turmoil to be in! I couldn't really stop what I was doing and I got myself into a really anxious state. Then I remembered the 'Act As If' I thought 'OK, I'll just act as if I'm fine, and go for it'. So I carried on, aware of how I was feeling, but acting as if I was fine and, of course, I got through it and everything was fine, as promised! When I spoke to a couple of the participants about it later in the week, they told me they had not noticed a thing.

I've used 'Act As If' in many situations and it has always helped me. I've used it to act as if I'm strong and powerful when walking down a dark street at night; I've used it in social situations when I've been unsure of myself; I've used it to act as if I've had lots of sleep when, in fact, I've only had a couple of hours.

Pause now for a moment if you want to, and think about times when 'Act As If' might be a useful thing for you to do. You could make a note in your journal.

Here is a lovely quote to end this chapter (if the word 'God' does not resonate with you, you might substitute 'Spirit' or 'The Universe').

You are a child of God. Your playing small does not serve the world. There is nothing enlightened about shrinking so that other people won't feel insecure about you. We were born to manifest the glory of God that is within us

Nelson Rockefeller

Chapter 10

Take Charge

"If you do not change direction,
you may end up where you are heading "
Lao Tzu, Chinese Taoist Philosopher

Sometimes I get scared by those highly motivated individuals – professional motivational speakers – who advise us to live life at maximum speed and intensity, who tell us to write goals and take massive action. In a way, I resent their drive, focus and intensity and yet ... they do have a point. For a start, it is really useful to have some idea of personal direction. Life is certainly easier if you know where you are heading. Just knowing which way to face is a dilemma solved! When your menopause starts, it can feel as if you are no longer in charge of yourself. Some people say they just don't feel like themselves any more. Maybe we are no longer quite who we once were, and it's perhaps time to change direction or confirm that we are on the right track.

Do you know what I mean when I say that at times I feel like I am in the driving seat of my life, and at other times it's as if my life is driving me? Occasionally, I feel as if I'm not even in the car! I'm behind the car, in a trailer, looking behind and paying no attention, with no idea where I am heading! Someone once said to me they felt they were in the boot and didn't want to come out. This chapter is about setting your own direction, creating the map of where you want to go, taking your place behind the wheel and setting off. Jump in, get in gear, stick your foot on the accelerator and let's go!

But first of all we need to: Stop. Think about where you are going and take charge of yourself and the journey. Work out your direction and then do what it takes to get you there. Whoops, I'm in danger of talking like one of those motivational people I mentioned before! But it's really no different from any other thing that you decide to do something about, such as clearing out a cupboard, organising your filing or making dinner. The process is the same: you work out your desired end result and do the actions to get what you want. You don't stop and look at it, see how it feels, talk to other people about it or complain about how awful it is. No. You think it through and just get on with it. So what about using that same way of thinking with the menopause and how you might be affected by it? Being proactive rather than reactive.

By the way, I'm not suggesting that everyone has taken the approach that I have described here, that's probably just me! I started with a 'wait and see' policy. I didn't do anything after my initial visits to the doctor – I thought it would go away by itself, that the symptoms would sort themselves out. I was also unsure as to what was actually a menopause symptom as opposed to a symptom of something else. It's easy to blame everything that happens on a) ageing or b) the menopause. For example, I found myself being very, very tired. I would wake up in the morning after eight hours deep sleep, feeling exhausted and that I could do with another five hours. I was worn out, found it hard to get any energy throughout the day at all and I was ready for bed at 9 p.m. I assumed that it was a menopausal symptom. Then I visited a homeopathic doctor who suggested I cut out wheat and cow's milk products for three weeks. Initially that was really hard to do. I love bread so much, I craved it because I felt it would give me energy but, in fact, the opposite was true. The more wheat I ate, the more my energy levels would drop. I persevered and was surprised at how much wheat is lurking in everyday products. The biggest surprise is that there is wheat in soy sauce – who would have thought! Anyway, I stuck with it and, to my delight, within five days I felt like a completely new person: lots of energy, sleeping well, and lost a couple of pounds to boot! Wonderful!

That was when I decided to take action, try things and see what I could do to make things better. Thinking about yourself, what could you do?

Some people are motivated by goals, love to write lists, get things done, make decisions and move on. You can recognise these people by their promptness; they like to be on time. They love to be organised so you will typically see a really tidy and ordered home/desk/garage. They always like to have a plan so they know what they are doing at the weekend. They start their Christmas shopping in September, or even before; they DO NOT leave it until the last minute.

Other people prefer to keep their options open, they like to spot new opportunities, they *don't* like to make decisions and prefer to leave things until the last minute. They are often motivated by fast-approaching, towering deadlines. You can recognise them by their flexible attitude to time or, in other words, a tendency to be late! They like to live life in the moment, taking opportunities as they come.

As you might expect, goal-setting works really well for the first group and not quite so well for the second group who often find it tricky to decide which goals to aim for. By the way, both have the ability to achieve things and hit deadlines, it's just that they go about it in completely different ways.

Think about your own preference and reflect on how you currently approach things you want to achieve. Do you prefer to make decisions and move on, or do you prefer to keep your options open? How proactive are you? What is your attitude? As we go through this chapter, collect the information that you need to plan and chart your journey through the multifaceted waters of the menopause.

Attitude

The way I see it, you have a choice: either you run your menopause, or it runs you. Now I know there are lots of elements which we cannot necessarily control, like bleeding or hormonal changes, but we can change our attitude to what happens.

Epictetus the Greek philosopher said: *People are not disturbed by things, but by the view they take of them.*

It's not what happens to you that matters, it's your attitude and perspective that makes the difference. Depending on our point of view, we can make a sunny day miserable and a wet day a thoroughly brilliant experience.

From my research, here are examples of both positive and negative attitude.

Gill told me, "The story I remember which resonates for me is a lady on my coaching course who said she 'didn't do the menopause.' I remember feeling the same way about morning sickness when I was pregnant and never experienced it". Her best advice was, "Use mind over matter and, if that doesn't work, go to a Homeopath".

Someone else told me, "I feel like an old, worn out hag which is what I never wanted to be. I never wanted to be a mean old Moaning Minnie, but that is what I have become."

Just pause for a moment and think about what your attitude is to the menopause, how you feel about it, what you notice, and also what you say to yourself.

Here's the sort of thing I mean. The other day I was making some lunch. I got a plate out of the cupboard; the plate was dirty, covered in crumbs. Since I knew that I had been the last person to tidy, I knew that I had put it there rather than in the dishwasher. The first thought that sprang, unbidden and completely unwelcome, into my head was 'Oh well, I expect that's just another sign of me getting old'. NO! STOP! Do not say that sort of thing to yourself!

Remember we get what we focus on, so if I'm focusing on 'signs I'm getting older' then that is what I filter for, that is what I see and that is what I begin to create and nurture and grow over time. What a shock to hear myself saying that. So, to remedy the situation, the trick is to decide what you are going to replace the negative thought with. For me it was 'That's really silly, it's got nothing to do with old age, it's just a simple error; when I was 15 I made simple errors, too'. My advice is not to age yourself prematurely with careless self-talk. My husband used to say things like, 'Now that I'm getting on a bit' or 'Oh, that's happened because I'm an old man now'. He meant it as a joke, but he was only 52 at the time, far too young to even be beginning to think about himself an old man. Fortunately, he stopped doing it when I explained the possible consequences to him.

Listen carefully to the things you say *about* yourself, and the things you say *to* yourself. When I was learning NLP, I remember the trainer saying that our unconscious mind does not have a sense of humour; it takes everything at face value and delivers to us what we think about or say. Have you noticed the people who make jokes at their own expense, to amuse other people? The sad thing is that often others don't find it particularly humorous. Then there are those who put themselves down saying things like, 'I'm useless at this' or 'I'm hopeless at that'. These negative messages give direct instructions to our unconscious mind, which is doing its best to bring into reality what we think about and therefore wish for. This idea of 'you get what you focus on' is wonderful when used in a positive way e.g. when we talk about people manifesting what they want. But the same concept can also deliver negatives if that is what we give attention to. So make sure you focus on what you want.

Motivation

Knowing how you are motivated and how you motivate yourself is another important factor if you are going to take charge of how you feel about the menopause.

You might find it interesting to recognise whether your motivation pattern is either Towards or Away From, also known as the Pain versus Pleasure principle; essentially it is the 'carrot or stick' approach.

People who are motivated Towards are stimulated by positive things, moving towards pleasure. If they have a goal they are working towards, they will focus on the positive outcome and all the benefits they will get from achieving that goal. These benefits will drive them to take action; they go for the carrot.

People who have Away From motivation are driven to act to get away from pain. If there is a goal they want to achieve, they will tend to focus on the negative consequences of not getting what they want and they will be driven to act by avoiding the bad stuff. They want to get away from the stick.

People can be motivated by one or the other of these motivation patterns or they may have a combination of the two. For me, I have a 50/50 mixture of the two. Some people may be Towards with some Away From, or Away From with some Towards.

Example:

A person begins to get hot flushes and decides she needs to do something about it, find out what she can do to alleviate the symptoms. Here's how she would express the situation, depending on the motivation pattern.

The Towards person:	I'm going to do something about this so that I can feel better, be comfortable and improve my well-being.
The Away From person:	I've got to do something about this, I'm fed up of feeling this way, and I've got to stop this getting worse.
Towards and Away From:	I want to do something about this, I want to feel better and I've got to stop these awful symptoms.
Away from and Towards:	I'm so fed up with these hot flushes, they are becoming more and more frequent. I'm going to find out how I can improve the situation and make myself feel better.

Stop and think for a minute about how you are motivated:

- Do you focus on the positives and go for it?

- Do you wait until things get too bad and then do something about it?

- Or do you do a mix of the two?

You can increase your motivation quite easily, by amplifying whichever one motivates you:

- If you are Towards motivated then find as many benefits and reasons as you can for taking action i.e. add more carrots

- If you are Away From motivated, find as many negative consequences as you can to propel you out of the 'stick zone' into taking action i.e. get more and bigger sticks

- If you are a bit of both, then do both, more carrots and more sticks!

If you have a tendency to the Away From pattern, practise more focusing on the positive, for a very simple reason: it's better for you. It's better for your mood, for your health and for the people around you.

So, as you are taking charge of yourself and your life, to help you to focus on the positives and use this towards motivation, here is an activity you can do. It is really useful to have your ideas represented in a visual way, you can add to it when you want and you can use it to help you keep up your momentum. It will also be really useful to help you focus on days when your motivation is not so high. I call it 'My Future Board'. This is a way of capturing all the positive things you want to focus on that you can look at when your motivation is not so high.

My Future Board

It's really easy, fun and relaxing to do. You'll need some artist's board or a large piece of card, ideally A3 sort of size, some glue, scissors and magazines with pictures. Then you create a collage representing the life you want, cutting out images that represent what you want and gluing them on your board.

You might be thinking that this all sounds too much trouble and that you don't have the time or the energy to do this sort of thing. However, it is really worth the effort. It's an activity that engages both sides of the brain and helps you to be creative. Plus, if you don't do it, you'll never know what you might be missing by way of a resource to help you in challenging times; also you might miss an opportunity to find out more about who you are and what you want in your life. Afterwards you can judge whether it was a good idea or not, but give it a go, there is nothing to lose and everything to gain.

If you cannot do it right now, you could make a plan for when would be a good time. Give it a go and engage your conscious and unconscious mind in creating the new life you want.

If the above activity really is 'a leap too far' then this next activity might suit you better. It is meant to help you to consider what you have already achieved, what you want to do more of/ less of and what you love to do/hate to do.

Alternative activity

For this you just need pen and paper or your journal and some free time.

Ask yourself these questions:

What have I achieved, what have I done already that I am pleased, proud and happy with?

What do I want to do more of?

What do I want to do less of or stop doing?

What do I love to do?

What do I hate to do?

If this is it, before the end of my life, what do I want to make sure I have achieved/done?

This is your life, to do with as you please, to do what you want to do. Take charge; take responsibility for it and for yourself. If you haven't done so already, let go of blaming circumstances or other people and bemoaning the situation. Free yourself so you can start to build the life you really want!

Chapter 11

Look after yourself

"And remember, no matter where you go, there you are."
Confucius

The menopause is a time of big change for us, our bodies are not quite the same and, for some of us, our minds don't seem to function quite the same either. How we react to that can take up a lot of energy and, for some, it can all be quite stressful. I find that it can destabilise me and put me off my stride. On some days I can't find my words or where I've put things, yet on other days I feel absolutely fine. On some days I have hot flushes and barely notice them; on other days they really knock me for six. On some days I feel physically drained; on others I'm full of energy and ready for anything.

I did have a tendency to get annoyed and frustrated with myself when I wasn't on top form, but I'm learning to give myself a break. I need to be my own best supporter and friend while I'm going through these times. So when I feel tired or not at my best, I give myself some time and space to recharge my batteries. This is not merely being self-indulgent; this is an absolute must if I want to stay in good shape mentally, physically and emotionally.

I still have a faint residue of guilt in the back of my mind when I take it easy, but I know that I need to take that time to look after myself.

This chapter is about taking good care of YOU, physically and emotionally. Nurturing, cherishing and loving yourself, for your own good and also for the people around you. (For those people who feel it is really not OK to be selfish, let me remind you that if you don't look after yourself well, you will not be in a good position to look after others.)

Look after yourself: Physically

We are surrounded by messages about what to eat and what not to eat, products that will make us look beautiful, exercise advice. It can be completely confusing and overwhelming. How many diets have I tried over my life? I've lost count: lots of carbohydrates, no carbohydrates, only protein, only fruit, masses of vegetables, weighing out portions, calorie-counting, pre-prepared foods. The list goes on and on.

On a day-to-day basis, we are bombarded with advertising, magazine articles and headlines about losing weight to look good, how to look younger without surgery (or with surgery). Whilst looking your best and maintaining a healthy body weight is a really good thing to do, there is an underlying presupposition that:

+ We are not OK as we are

+ Looking good = being thin + being young

I have always been prone to being overweight and I now wonder whether that was just a belief fuelled by the messages in the media and the diet industry. Hmmm ... something to think about.

They say that women have a tendency to gain weight around the time of the menopause. Sometimes I agree with this and sometimes I don't. I have two different stories that I can tell to illustrate that, from the past few years.

Story 1

In 2006, I went to the gym every other day, this included one session per week with a personal trainer. I followed a diet from what I considered to be the best diet book ever for me (more on that shortly) and followed five simple rules:

1. *Exercise regularly*

2. *Drink lots of water*

3. *Cut out cappuccinos and fancy coffee*

4. *Cut out alcohol on weekdays and only drink it at the weekend*

5. *Cut out bread*

Result: I looked great; I felt fantastic and lost about 14lbs

Story 2

In 2007, I would 'try' to go to the gym three times a week but, in reality, I maybe went once a week. I shifted from the personal trainer to Pilates (thereby missing my cardio-vascular exercise which got my heart rate up). I dropped the five simple rules and ate whatever I felt like. I was 'too busy' in the last three months to go to the gym or exercise regularly.

Result: I felt sluggish, I looked lumpy and gained 12lbs

Now, if you had asked me in 2007, I could easily have blamed the menopause for the fact that I had gained weight. Looking back, I wouldn't have thought to mention that I'd been out for dinner at least once, nearly every week. Nor would I have reported that I'd had a starter and a main course and maybe even pudding, too. And another thing: for a little while, I got into the habit of finishing at the gym and then going to one of those coffee places and ordering a chai tea latte – of course not a single calorie in those! Hah! I've since discovered it's around 200 calories for a medium-size one!! Why not just have a Mars Bar and be done with it! It's not surprising, is it, that I gained weight? I could blame it on the menopause if I wanted to, but who's kidding who?

Note: you might be thinking that the gym is not for you and that you would do something different. That's great, now all you need to do is work out what that something different is and make it something that you can and will enjoy. You probably know as well as I do that exercise is really good for you, helps to make you feel happier by releasing endorphins and will also help you to be more agile and fit for your later years. So have a think.

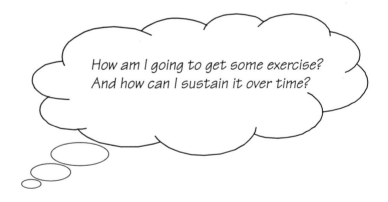

Exercise

In the gym or somewhere else, it's really worth finding at least one activity which gets you moving that you enjoy. Swim, walk, Salsa dancing, fencing, Wii Fit, following a video at home – do something, it will help you keep your waist! If you don't, in 10 years time you might be thinking 'I wish I had exercised more when I was younger'. It's pretty much guaranteed that you won't be wishing that you had spent more time sitting watching TV!)

Remember just a ten-minute walk every day is better than nothing.

Right now you are creating your body for the rest of your life. What you feed it, how you take care of it, and whatever you do now, will be reflected in how you feel and look in future years. Are you sure you are doing enough for it?

Eat well

Find your own way, a way that works for you. What I have also discovered for myself over the last five years is this: every person's body and metabolism is different, therefore following one-size-fits-all diets designed for everyone does not work. I mentioned my favourite diet book: it is *The Metabolic Typing Diet* by William L. Wolcott and Trish Fahey. This book teaches you about finding your own personal fuel mix so that your body works at its optimum. We all have different and specific Carbohydrate and Protein mixes; when you discover your own, you should find you have a lot more energy and feel better.

I am trying out the Hay system just now, where you don't mix carbohydrate and protein at the same meal. I'm loving it, my digestion seems better, I've lost a few pounds and I have lots more energy.

The main point is: experiment; find what works for you, not necessarily what the diet industry tells you, but what you know works for your body and yourself.

I was at a grand dinner a few weeks ago; one of the ladies was complaining about how she just could not lose weight, she had tried absolutely everything but nothing worked. A little while later, she asked my husband if he was going to eat the potatoes he had left on his plate, then she scoffed those as well as her own! She is not alone; lots of people don't notice or forget where they might be over-indulging, or they tell themselves that they eat like sparrows when, in actual fact, they are eating for an entire flock!

Our metabolism tends to slow a little as we grow older, and we might be getting a bit less exercise – it only takes one or two extra chips a day to mount up to an extra 14lbs over the course of a year.

Experiment with keeping a food diary. This is a really good activity to do because we don't always realise exactly how much we take in; we forget the odd slice of toast or biscuit or glass of wine. It can be easy to kid ourselves that we are eating less than we really are. By writing everything you eat in a food diary, you can get real about what you are consuming, and then you can make decisions about how to adjust your intake to suit yourself. It is important to be honest, though

Also in your food diary write about what your beliefs are about diet and food and you.

Note: for some people the word 'diet' has negative associations; if that is so for you, try to find a different word that works better, like 'plan' or 'regime'.

Rest, Relaxation and Sleep

As your body re-balances itself in its new state, make sure you do get enough rest to allow your body to restore itself. If you want to, you could allow yourself a cat-nap or a power nap (though not too much sleep during the day, or you could end up not being able to sleep at night). If you have trouble sleeping, you might try keeping a sleep diary, making a note of how long you sleep for, when you wake up, what your emotional state was at bedtime, what you ate and drank the evening before. You'll be able to track how much sleep you get and also check if there are any patterns of behaviour that you can change. Take time for yourself and relax when you can.

Physical Space

Now turn your attention to your environment. Are you comfortable in your home? Does it support you and help you to maintain a happy and healthy life? Take a fresh look at your surroundings. It's easy to get so familiar with things that we no longer notice that we are not quite content with them.

Coming up next is something you can do in this area: this is about looking at your home and evaluating how it looks, feels, sounds and smells. This is an element of your life where you do have control; you can make an instant impact, even by making some small changes. The benefits are that it will give you a new perspective on your home, you can discover how to change your environment to suit yourself and you will end up with a home environment that works, fits for you and complements your lifestyle.

How it can make you feel

You choose how much you want to do in each area; it's up to you whether you want to just move a lamp or a cushion, or whether you have a mind to completely refurbish. Do a room a day, a week, a month or a year, whatever works for you and depending on how much time, money and energy you have.

The smallest of changes can make a big difference. For example reorganising a book-case that has been getting on your nerves, or relocating a potted plant.

Whether you feel there is a lot to do or a little, do it in your own time. The purpose is to improve your physical space and environment. Start with the room where you spend the most time and go on from there.

Clear your space - Decorate - Enjoy!

Activity – Assessing your environment

Time required: up to you, you decide how much time you want to spend

Kit: pen and paper or notebook

Take one room or space in your home. Go into that room and look at it as if you have never seen it before and assess it as if it belonged to someone else, or you were looking at it through someone else's eyes. Check for the following:

If you want to, you can score them out of ten, or make a mark on the line

	0 Low		10 High

Comfort:

Furniture:

Soft furnishings:

Decor:

How much do I like
being in this room:

What are the things you love about this room?

What clutter can you remove?

What things are redundant?

What do you want to change?

What's missing?

Now make a plan: to make improvements over the next six months to a year as you see fit. Keep it simple and achievable and do something every day to reach your goal. Even if you only have energy and time to do one tiny action, do that. Not only does it signal to your unconscious mind that this is something important, it is also keeping a commitment to yourself, and you will be finished all the sooner; plus you will get a daily sense of satisfaction.

You may want to discuss this with the other people you live with ☺

Use your journal to reflect on the process and notice what you are learning and discovering about yourself and how you like to live.

Balance

Take a good long look at your life and work out whether you are in balance.

Are you out of balance, feeling frazzled, struggling to fit everything in and having no time for yourself? Are you enjoying your life, spending time doing what you love doing, making enough space for the things that are important to you?

Remember also that what worked for you five years or two years or even six months ago may not work for you now. Take a fresh look at things and make your diagnosis. Now you can decide what you are going to do about it, write it down so that you don't forget, and take action. I suggest you keep a special space in your journal for this; you can signpost it with a sticky label or a tab. I also recommend writing these actions on post-it notes and sprinkling them liberally around you to remind you of your intention.

Look after yourself: Mentally

Many women describe symptoms of being fuzzy-headed and not being able to concentrate so well.

The brain is like a muscle: use it or you lose it! It's easy to go through life in automatic, doing what you usually do, eating the same sort of things, watching the same TV programmes. I'd like to introduce you to the way I see it: the paradox of the human brain (remember I'm not a scientist!).

On the one hand, we love to learn, we like new things, we like to discover things; in a way we are like learning machines. In fact, sometimes we can't help ourselves from learning. We pick up information from newspapers, books, TV, friends, everywhere – and we collect it and store it, and we use that information to update what we do and what we think. It's amazing and it's automatic.

On the other hand, as human beings we are creatures of habit. We look for patterns to follow, we have the ability to work out how to do something and then we take the path of least resistance and do the same thing every time. For example, most people have the same breakfast every day or go to work the same way every day.

Now this is a wonderful ability, it means that we can work out how to do something, create our mental 'computer programme' and then, when it is time to do that thing, it's as if we can press a 'go' button and the programme runs automatically. Brilliant, we can do loads of stuff without thinking about it, like emptying the dishwasher. Do you think about it? Probably not. Most likely, you've devised a practical way to do it that works for you. Here's mine:

1. Open dishwasher

2. Pull out bottom rack, put away pots and pans, then big plates, followed by small plates, then bowls

3. Pull out top rack , put away mugs then glasses

4. Take out cutlery basket and put away cutlery: knives, spoons, forks, teaspoons

5. Then put away anything else that is left in there

My husband always turns the machine off when he opens the door (on/off switch is in the top of the door).

My sister has added a step: she pats dry the bases of the cups and glasses with a tea towel after she has pulled the top rack out. No more dripping water everywhere. Genius! Why didn't I think of that? Because I was operating in automatic mode.

These two additions (switch off and pat dry) would really improve my dishwasher-emptying skills; however, because I'm running my usual programme, I forget to add them.

If I want to perfect my skills, I would need to practise consciously until I remembered to do it right every time. They say it takes 28 days to create a habit, so that's how long I would need to practise for. The new programme would look like this:

1.   Open dishwasher – *switch it off*

2.   Pull out bottom rack, put away pots and pans, then big plates, followed by small plates, then bowls

3.   Pull out top rack, pat *the bases of mugs and glasses with a tea towel* then put them away

4.   Take out cutlery basket and put away cutlery: knives, spoons, forks, teaspoons

5.   Then put away anything else that is left in there

It's possible that there are many different and better ways of emptying a dishwasher (or any other task I might want to do) but as long as I'm in automatic, I'm not thinking about what I'm doing, never mind whether I can do anything to improve things.

How this relates to those of us steaming through the menopause is that we could be 'in automatic' when maybe we could improve things by stopping and thinking, using our brains to make our world a better place, and creating a happier, easier environment… or at least get the most efficient dishwasher-emptying programme!

(If you don't have a dishwasher, you can construct an example for yourself, perhaps based on unpacking the grocery shopping and putting it away – think about the habitual process you use, the steps that you follow every time without thinking.)

Pause for a moment and consider other times when you are in automatic and could use some improvement.

Think

Could it be that there are areas of your life that you have
been ignoring or not noticing? Is there some part where you
pretend everything is fine, even though it really is not?

I remember once sitting with a friend having a glass of
wine and chatting about our lives and how we were. He said
to me, "But you have a nice life, don't you?" In that moment
when I thought about it, I had the trappings of a nice life:
a relationship of 13 years with a good man, a lovely six-
bedroomed house with a paddock in the countryside with
views to die for, a house in the South-west of France that we
went to frequently, a beautiful spaniel, a great job doing what
I love, working with wonderful people. What more could I ask
for? And yet I was lonely in the relationship and unhappy with
myself. All this came to my mind as I looked for the answer to
his question and, to my surprise, out came the response, "No,
actually, I don't have a nice life because I am not happy in it".
Deep inside I knew I was not happy, but it was another thing
to actually verbalise it because, once I had said it out loud, it
became a *thing* that I had to do something about, rather than
a thought I could ignore.

• Do yourself a favour: think, reflect, muse and contemplate
  and use your journal to exercise your brain by thinking
  differently about things

• Evaluate how you are using your time: for example you
  could check that you are not watching too much TV; it's
  easy to get sucked into a habit of watching programmes
  for the sake of it, either because we are in automatic, or
  because we don't bother to think of something else to do. If
  that is the case, perhaps experiment and have a television-
  free day and see what happens

• Get your brain working; it's like a muscle, we have to
  keep using it to keep it strong and agile. You can try brain

exercises like puzzles, crosswords or Sudoku. There are also games and brain-training exercises that you can use on small handheld devices and on the internet.

• Learn something new like bridge or aromatherapy

• Learn a poem or just practise remembering your shopping list

Be creative about how you can get your brain operating at full stretch.

Already, if you are taking more exercise, beautifying, de-cluttering and organising your environment and exercising your brain, you will find your head becoming clearer. It's also important to notice what you focus on.

Happiness is a choice

You can choose to focus on the things that make you happy, or otherwise. Notice for yourself where your attention tends to go: to the positive or the negative. Here's a story about someone I know to illustrate what I mean.

Shirley spends her life focusing on the things she doesn't like, on what is wrong with the world and she often finds fault with other people. She is wary of everyone and worries about how others see her. When things are going well, she thinks it is too good to be true and that it can't last. She went on holiday with a friend; when they came back and were describing how it was, Shirley said that she had had quite a good time, described how she liked the architecture and a meal out that they had both enjoyed. She then went on to complain about the hotel, the flight, the service on one day at breakfast and on and on. By the time she had finished, she had taken all the pleasure out of the experience by focusing on the negative. Later on I spoke to her friend Jean, who was the sort of person who always focuses on the positive. Jean had a fantastic time, she described meeting some lovely people, she had enjoyed the cuisine and loved the city with its impressive buildings and interesting shops. They both went to the same place and had a completely different experience because of what they chose to focus on.

Overwhelm: clarity and priorities

Some women experience 'brain fuzziness' at this time of life, but menopause might not be the only cause. It could also come from just having too much to on your plate, or trying to do too much, which can lead to feeling overwhelmed. Stress and overwhelm come hand in hand. We get anxious and lose the ability to focus. In that state we are unable to think clearly. It's like having lots of yellow post-it notes flying round in your head with no glue on them and nowhere to stick them! The fight or flight response is triggered, our brain function shifts to emergency mode and we find it really hard to think and to cope.

Three things you can do to get out of that feeling of Overwhelm:

1. Stop trying to do **everything**. Pause and take 10 long, slow breaths, in through the nose and out through the mouth. This will reset your system.

2. Next, write down everything that is on your mind (usually you'll find it's not as much or as bad as you think).

3. Then prioritise. Part of the problem is usually that you are trying to think about and do lots of things at the same time. No matter how great at multi-tasking you are, you can actually only really do *one* thing at a time, in the moment. Look at your list and decide: if I only did three of these, which would I do? Then you can do those three things; if there's time, you can do some more.

Also check your list for things 'not to do'; maybe some items are so far down your list of priorities that you are *never* really going to get round to them. Give yourself a break and just let go of them, and let go also of the pressure you put on yourself to achieve.

These three steps enable you to step out of the emotion and help you to get your brain back on track and give you some control. Once you recognise what you are dealing with, then you can handle things much more easily.

Another idea to exercise your brain is to ask yourself:

'What are the important things in my life that are just not getting done, that I am not paying attention to or that I can't seem to find the time for?' Then write down as many ways as possible that you could actually make those things happen. What actions could you take?

Engaging the help of professionals

One of the options you might come up with is to get some help; you don't have to do it alone. You could ask a friend or you could go to a professional. Some experts you could think of turning to would be:

Homeopath

Coach

Nutritionist

Therapist

Hypnotherapist

Acupuncturist

NLP practitioner

Massage therapist

You could also try Reiki, Reflexology, Thought Field Therapy – there are many therapies that you might find helpful.

Nurture yourself

Here are some ideas of things you might like to do. The list is obviously not exhaustive. You can add to it to make it even longer, and then refine it to include only your favourites.

Some of the things on the list you will like the sound of and some not, just choose the ones that are for you but do consider trying out those that appeal to you least. You might discover something that you didn't realise you liked and now you do! Who knows what changes we will find for ourselves in the menopause?

Most of the items on the list are free, illustrating that you don't necessarily need money to spend time for yourself and your well-being.

admire a tree

be grateful

dog walk

drink something delicious: tea, wine, champagne

eat something you love, maybe chocolate or a juicy piece of fruit

get lost in nature

get moving

get up early and enjoy the peace

go barefoot

listen to a favourite piece of music

look at photos and enjoy being nostalgic

meditate

read a magazine

read a poem

sing to yourself

smell some favourite fragrances

stay an extra hour in bed and luxuriate

stop and listen to the world outside

take 10 minutes to simply be – do nothing

take a bubble bath

watch clouds

write a letter

write a poem

Make your own list in your journal, aim to collect at least 72, and add to your list when you find something else you like. If you highlight these pages in your journal with a sticky label or a sticky tab, you'll be able to find them easily at a later date when you feel like nurturing yourself.

Let yourself relax

Give yourself permission to switch off for a while, and think of this as a necessity rather than a luxury. Whether you take a five-minute holiday in your head, or go and lie under a tree in a park or garden for two hours, work out how you can get yourself to relax. What is it that relaxes you?

a warm bath?

an episode of your favourite soap opera?

a favourite CD?

a beautiful picture?

Now that we are at the end of this chapter, why not take a few minutes to yourself to just relax and let the world drift by outside of you.

See you on the next page when you are done!

Chapter 12

What about work

72% of menopausal women work either full- or part-time

78% of those women say their symptoms affect them at work

93% say they couldn't discuss the menopause with their boss

73% say they can't discuss their symptoms with work colleagues

In this chapter we look at problems you might encounter at work as a result of the menopause, what you can do about it and how to make a plan of action to deal with it.

Menopausal or Perimenopausal, it is definitely worth taking time to think about how it might affect your work, and planning how you want to manage yourself in the workplace. Even if you are the sort of person who is mostly sailing through this life stage, you may still find it useful to take stock of where you are and plan for the next phase. Some of the areas where women have found the menopause affecting them at work are:

Performance: changes in concentration levels and fuzzy thinking can affect our ability to think and to make decisions. Some people find it more of a challenge to handle the multiple demands of a busy role.

Relationships: some women say that they feel a separation from other colleagues; they feel reluctant to bring up the subject of the menopause in case the other person looks upon it negatively, or might tease them. There is also a concern that bringing up this subject, which is alien to the other person, creates a gulf in the relationship that previously was not there.

Motivation: tiredness can decrease our motivation level. Some people find that things which were previously highly important to them change at this time of life. Others might question where they work and what they are doing, for example whether they really want to be in a fast-paced corporate environment or whether they could be doing something else that would make them feel happier.

Self perception: the menopause brings with it a new sense of identity where we learn and discover how this new self fits into our current environment. Where previously we would not have given it a moment's thought, we consciously start to think about who we are and who we want to be in the world of work.

Energy levels: some of us don't have the same energy and physical stamina that we had twenty years previously. For me, this realisation has come as an unwelcome visitor. I had always been used to having the physical strength to do most things that I wanted to do, and an amazing ability to keep going until the job was done. What I notice now is that I can still do those things but it takes me longer to recover. In the past, if I had a tough week of both work and play, I'd have a lie-in on a Saturday and I would feel fine by Sunday. Now I find that it takes me all weekend to recover, and maybe even into the following week.

Here are some other examples of how it affects women at work:

Jenny tells me that she has been used to being an attractive blonde in a young and dynamic company. She then finds herself shocked to discover that she does not get noticed as much as she did previously, finding it hard to get attention. She dreads the hot flushes. She is 45.

Sarah has noticed that her previously full head of hair is thinner than it was, her waist has thickened a little and she is worried that people will be thinking of her as old and is concerned how that will affect her career. She is 47.

Liz is stressed out, she's feels as if she is running herself ragged. She says her thinking is foggy and she does not feel the same clarity that she used to feel in meetings. She missed an important meeting because somehow it wasn't in her diary. She feels scared and insecure as she feels she is not her normal self. She is 51.

Jude completely lost her temper in a team meeting, she raged and ranted at her staff because they missed a key piece of information out of a report. Even as she was doing it, she knew it was a 'bad idea' but couldn't seem to stop. She is 49.

These are examples of women who are finding it tricky to navigate the waters of work whilst at the same time experiencing some of the features of the menopause. Of course, there is no one-size-fits-all solution. It's best if you find the way that works for you, working out the challenges you yourself have to overcome and working out how you are going to do that.

You need to be in charge, rather than the menopause running you or sidetracking your behaviour. It is vital to get a grip and decide how you might handle any symptoms you are having, even though we know that some of these are not necessarily under your immediate control. I have several coaching clients who have decided to take the time to work on themselves. Together we explore how this affects their work identity, what their long-term plan is and what changes they would like to make. We have also generated practical strategies for dealing with their individual symptoms. They have all said how much it helps to talk to someone about this, outside of their work environment. There is a great deal of value to be had by getting some support and some help in this area, particularly because, for most women, it's not easy to talk to work colleagues or the boss about it. Even in our liberal and open society, it seems to be one of our great taboos, not many people talk about it openly. I have certainly noticed embarrassed faces when I have brought up the topic in conversation. The metaphor of the elephant in the room springs to mind: everyone knows it is there, it's something really big, but we all pretend that it isn't there. Perhaps if we ignore it, maybe it will go away.

I believe it's critical to get a handle on these issues to make sure you safeguard your work and your livelihood. If you want to get some control and find solutions for yourself, here is a technique you can use.

First things first: think about yourself and your situation at work and make a note of any symptoms that you want to be able to handle better. For me, it is fuzzy thinking and forgetfulness.

Technique: The GROW model

This is a great coaching tool. It's called GROW which stands for Goal. Reality, Options and Will, from Sir John Whitmore's book Coaching for Performance. In coaching, we use it for goal-setting and solving problems. Here we use it to work out how to handle the issues and questions we are facing in the workplace as a result of menopausal symptoms or changes.

It is really simple, I thoroughly recommend it any time you have a challenge you need to deal with. The GROW model has four steps, as follows:

G = GOAL

Having identified the problem or the challenge that you face, what is your goal in relation to it? I might be tempted to say something like, 'My goal is to not have hot flushes'. Whilst this might be exactly what I want, this is the wrong way to express it. Why? Because it means I am focusing on what *I don't want*, as opposed to what *I do want*. The way to do this is to ask yourself what you want instead. Phrase your goal in the positive. For example, if my goal is to not have hot flushes, asking, 'What do I want instead?' might elicit answers something like these:

> I want to minimise hot flushes

or

> I want to feel comfortable when I have a hot flush

or

> I want to deal easily with the embarrassment I feel at hot flushes

For me, the challenge I want to overcome is fuzzy thinking and forgetfulness, so my goal is 'I want to clear my mind and remember things that are important'.

As you can imagine, the way you express and phrase your goal will have a direct bearing on how you solve the problem and what actions you take, so do take the time to make sure you are clear on what your goal is, and that you have expressed it in the positive.

R = REALITY

This means: What is the current reality? How are things at the moment? How am I coping with things? What is the situation just now? What have I already done about this problem or challenge? You need to look at the situation honestly and dispassionately and be realistic about what is actually happening. For example, someone might say, "I have hot flushes all day long" when, in reality, they have four flushes in the morning, ten in the afternoon and maybe six in the evening.

So, for my example of fuzzy thinking and forgetfulness, here is the reality:

> I am not so clear in my thinking in some areas of work, usually when I have a lot to think about, and do not devote enough time

to the topic ... or when my motivation is low, for example if it is something I don't want to do or I don't feel is important. I tidy things away and don't remember where I have put them because I am not concentrating on what I am doing. I have misplaced letters and receipts because I don't have a proper system for filing them.

O = OPTIONS

At this stage, you look at all the options that are available to you. Brainstorm as many as you can, get creative, add in any whacky or unusual ideas – at this stage it is just a case of thinking of all the possible things you could do. The more the merrier!

I once attended a course where the facilitator said, "There are 37 solutions to every problem". 'How marvellous,' I thought. 'Gosh, and I had just been looking for one solution! Now that I know there are 37, it makes it so much easier because, in actual fact, I probably only need *one* solution, but it's great to know that there are so many others out there. Having the belief that there are so many solutions to every problem also makes the problem feel easier to deal with. The next problem, of course, will be which of the 37 solutions to choose!'

I wonder how you would approach any problems you face at work if you knew that there were so many possible solutions. How wonderful to know that there are so many answers and you only have to find one or two of them.

(By the way, I don't know if there really are 37 solutions to every problem, I just find it a really useful belief to hold.)

So ... all of my possible options for the fuzzy thinking and forgetfulness:

1. Make list of priorities so that I know what is important

2. Write everything down that I have to do

3. Make a specific time for tidying so that I can concentrate on what I'm doing

4. Get a personal assistant

5. Get a Dictaphone and tell it what I want to do

6. Reduce the number of things I have on my mind

7. Organise my paper more effectively

8. Manage my diary better so that I have time to do admin tasks and also time to think

9. Do just one thing at a time – stop trying to multi-task ineffectively

10. Get a special notebook just for stuff that I want to remember

11. Let go of trying to remember to do everything, just do what I feel like

12. Change my diet; my head is clearer when I have not had carbohydrates

13. Make a note of how certain foods affect my thinking

14. Get more sleep; when I'm rested I think better

15. Track how my thinking might be different at different times of day and use what I discover to help me decide what to do when

16. Get a whiteboard so I can write things to remember on it

17. Ask someone else to remind me of the critical things

18. Make time to do something about the problem!

19. ... and

20. ... so

21. ... on

What you'll generally find is that if you keep asking 'What else could I do?' you will surprise yourself with the variety of responses and ideas you come up with.

Important: do not censor any of the ideas you come up with at this stage, accept them all and write them down. Even if you think it is a really rubbish idea, the next one that comes on the back of it might be a brilliant one.

W = WILL

This is the last step; now you look at your list of options, the things you *could* do, evaluate them all and decide what you actually *will do*. I suggest you pick out the key actions that will have the greatest impact and do those first. Don't just think about doing them; do them and then see what happens – you can track your progress in your journal.

So here is what I am going to do:

1. Set aside two hours on Wednesday morning this week to think about and do something about the problem

2. Write everything down that I have to do

3. Make a list of my top priorities so that I know what is important

4. Organise my papers and receipts more efficiently

5. Schedule time for admin tasks and also time to think

6. Make a note of how certain foods affect my thinking and change my diet; my head is clearer when I have not had carbohydrates

7. Get more sleep; when I'm rested I think better

Some comments from me on my list above:

Notice on my initial Options list, number 18, the last item was 'Make time to do something about the problem!'

When I put together my Do This List, it turns out that this has become the No 1 activity. It has been re-worded to be more specific and achievable.

Numbers 6 and 7 of my final list will be beneficial in many other areas of my life as well, so maybe I'll get two for the price of one!

As you can see, using the GROW model is a really easy way to coach yourself through a problem and to find practical and easy things that you can do to help yourself.

Managing your state

In general terms, this is about controlling how you feel, rising above what is currently going on for you, using your mind and body to help you to overcome emotions. Let me explain. The way we feel, the way we think and the way we hold our body are all interconnected. For example, if we feel down, we might drag our heels and if we are happy we tend to have a spring in our step. When we shift our thinking, we automatically shift our body posture.

Imagine Sally who is waiting for a telephone call to tell her whether she has been successful at an interview where she thinks she did pretty well. She is expecting the call at midday and she is really looking forward to speaking to the person. She prepares herself, with telephone, a pen and paper to hand. She's ready! But the telephone does not ring, it stays silent ... and stays silent for ages. She checks that it is still working and keeps on waiting – it's a very important call that she really doesn't want to miss. Her initial excitement at the beginning of the wait begins to fade, she starts to look and feel rather deflated. She begins to ask herself whether she had been kidding herself and that maybe she hadn't been that great at the interview after all. Her confidence dwindles, her shoulders sag and her head drops a little. That little voice in her head starts to berate her for being overconfident, telling her she was silly to expect to get the job. She then goes over the interview in her head, reviewing it and looking for reasons and proof that she was not really that good and she decides that they probably won't give her the job after all. She finds several questions which she now thinks she might have messed up. She torments herself with what she did wrong and what she could have done better. Her sparkle dulls and she resigns herself, with a sigh, and prepares herself for the disappointment ...

All that internal dialogue and self-doubt went on in her head, unprompted by any external stimulus of any sort. How our imagination can play tricks on us!

The telephone rings! Sally is startled out of her state of despondency ...

You can easily imagine this same situation and picture the main character experiencing many other different states of mind. The point is this: what we say to ourselves in our head affects how we feel; this in turn affects our body language, all of that affects our behaviour, which then influences what happens and the outcome we get.

The person in the story needs to manage their state, so that when the call finally does come, they are able to be in control, to handle and rise above their emotions.

The first step to doing this is to recognise, dispassionately, what is happening and to notice what and how we are thinking. This does involve listening to that little voice within, and paying attention to what it is saying. It doesn't necessarily mean that we give credence to that internal dialogue, just that we are aware of the content and the intent of the message.

The tricky bit is paying attention to the inner dialogue, and *at the same time* being present and staying with whatever is happening around you. The idea is not for you to go inside your head and do some 'in-the-moment psychoanalysis'; what you need to do is quickly note your thoughts and feelings and evaluate them in the light of the situation or the context that you find yourself in.

The next step is to decide, dispassionately, what you are going to do about the situation. This does involve some rather fancy multi-tasking! On the one hand, you are noticing your thoughts and feelings and deciding how to handle the situation; on the other hand, you are still relating and talking to the people around you.

Where I have found this incredibly useful is when I have been in meeting situations or in training situations when I was the centre of attention and a hot flush started. On the outside, I need to look confident and in control; on the inside, I'm asking myself things like, 'How long is this going to take, will they notice, I hope this is over soon, if I go red will they think I'm lying, will this trash my credibility?' etc. etc. If you are doubting your ability to do two things at once, it's likely that you've already been doing it, just maybe not in a conscious way. Rather than be sidetracked by hot flushes, just rise above it and work out how you are going to handle it.

More easily said than done? Give it a try and see how you get on.

... They ask for her by name. Time slows and seconds seem to take hours to pass. She listens but hardly hears when the voice says that they are calling following her interview, her mind races. Then she hears the words "Sally, we're delighted to offer you..."

Breathing

There are times when work can cause us to feel stressed and anxious. For example when there is too much to do, or when we are feeling more emotional than usual, the pressure is on and the deadlines are looming. These stresses, when coupled with hot sweats and fuzzy thinking, are a recipe for tension.

Another top tip for managing your state is to breathe, consciously. When we are relaxed, we breathe slowly, low down. You can put your hand on your tummy and feel the lower part of your ribcage and your stomach moving in and out as you breathe. When we are stressed, our breathing changes, the rate of breathing speeds up and we breathe more shallowly from the upper part of our chest. Have you ever noticed, when the stress is a shock, some people automatically put their open palm on the sternum? I remember a steward I worked with who nicknamed this surprise or shock gesture as a 'Hands on Pearls' moment! I did it on my wedding day, when I first saw my future husband standing waiting for me at the front of the room – it turned out to be one of his favourite photographs.

Of course, it's good to breathe! To manage your state, make sure you keep your breathing low and slow; that way you get maximum air intake to your brain, which allows you to think clearly. Practise shifting your breathing from low to high to low again, so that when you need to breathe low to calm yourself, it is easy and natural for you to do. How to practise: breathe all the way out and then breathe in again, filling the lower part of your lungs, which shifts your diaphragm down and pushes your tummy out. Take long, slow breaths, with the in-breath being the same length as the out-breath, for a slow count of four.

Note: If you are anything like me, when you are doing this don't be thinking about whether your tummy sticks out and you look fat! (only kidding)

Brand 'Me'

You might think of this as your corporate identity: how you look, how come across, your 'packaging'. This is about your image, which sends a message to colleagues and the organisation.

When you walk in the room, what does your image say about you? Does it reflect who you are and what you want to say? Recently, I went to see a client at their corporate offices who was telling me about a new senior member of the executive team. She told me about this new Director and then went on to give a detailed description of her style of clothing and hair, which was described as being 'stuck in the eighties'. Later, in separate conversations with two other people, the Director was mentioned again. They, too, had been similarly struck by the person's appearance. I'm not saying it's right or wrong, but it is a fact that people often judge a book by its cover, deciding what is on the inside by looking at the outside. They never did mention her skills or experience.

One of my clients is working on how to shift how she is perceived in the organisation, from being friendly and enthusiastic to being more calm and 'stateswoman-like'. She is paying attention to how she dresses and her communications – both written and in person.

I had a lovely time reinventing myself at around the time of my 50th birthday. I changed my hair, changed my style of clothing and also changed my make-up and lipstick. None of it was particularly drastic or shocking but it did bring my look up-to-date. The benefits were that I received lots of lovely compliments from all sorts of people. I felt more in tune with the people around me, I felt more confident and I think I looked great. I think it is easy to be lazy and to have the same hairstyle for 20 years because it suited you once upon a time. But times change, fashion changes, and you change; so, as my mother would say when I was lagging behind as a child, "Do keep up!"

Some people find it really easy to make those changes themselves but there are also books to help you. You could give yourself a real treat and see an image and colour specialist who will really help you to look at yourself in a new and improved light. They show you the colours and styles that are the most flattering and work best for you. Department stores also have make-up specialists who will give you lots of new ideas about how to update your look.

Have a think about it … are you slightly old-fashioned, and could you bring yourself more up-to-date? Perhaps even changing an accessory or two can bring new life to your appearance.

Note: I am not suggesting that you dress in a really young way, or change for the sake of changing. What I propose is that you take some time out – by yourself, with a friend or with an expert – and refresh your wardrobe so that you feel good about yourself. Make the most of your assets. Perhaps even push the boundaries and do something different, just to see what happens. Be bold and have fun!

Managing your profile and improving your reputation

Once you have had a good think about 'Brand Me' and what you look like, sound like and feel like, you are then in a strong position to leverage your brand in the marketplace so that you are seen as an attractive and desirable proposition. This is the sort of language that gets used in some organisations; the workplace is often full of these types of buzzwords or business-speak. Some readers might be unfamiliar with these terms. Whilst this is not the vocabulary that we use on an everyday basis, nevertheless we might still want to address the underlying message which is 'putting your best foot forward'. It's all about making the most of yourself and selling yourself and your skills.

What I mean by the term 'managing your profile' is to promote your talents and abilities in the workplace, to sell your skills and present yourself in such a way that people want you on their team, so they see the value that you can bring to the job. Furthermore, if you agree with the opinion that women become invisible as they get older, then unquestionably you need to blow your own trumpet so that you get seen, your voice is heard and that you stand out. I remember my mother telling me, as I was starting my first job, to work hard and to do my best, then I would get noticed and, as she put it, 'get on and do well'. The reality these days, particularly with people working in virtual teams and matrix structures, is that people are so busy that they are unaware of whether you are doing a good job or a fabulous one. Sometimes we only get noticed when we have done something wrong! Many organisations have flawed performance management systems that don't pick up on how well people are doing. In this case, you have to promote yourself and show what you can do.

Here are six top tips:

1. Use the Three Chairs technique on page 53 to look at how your work is perceived by different people or different departments.

2. Develop and nurture your people network. Make a mind map of your current contacts, both professional and personal, and then look at areas where it would be helpful to get to know people.

3. Offer to help others and they might help you in return. I'm not saying you should expect them to automatically help you in return. My belief is that when I help someone out, I know that the favour is returned somehow, by someone, though not necessarily by the original person I helped.

4. Learn more about your field and get to be known as an expert, share your knowledge and expertise by helping others. That way they will see what a good job you can do and can recommend you to others.

5. Tell people when you have done a good job. Some people feel really uncomfortable about doing this because it sounds too much like showing off. This is something of a British trait that many other cultures don't share. If you are reluctant to blow your own trumpet, here are a couple of alternative ways of looking at it and thinking about it:

   • If you are not prepared to speak about the things you are good at, and promote yourself, then you might miss a promotion because nobody knows about you or your skills and abilities

   • We like to hear about other people's successes as they can inspire our own. Therefore, talking about what you do well can have a positive effect on others

- Often we don't value our strengths because we mistakenly assume that *everyone* can do the things that we find easy. This is not the case; you are able to do things easily that others find difficult. When you promote your talents, it means that others can find the ideal person they need to do the best job

6. Take on a high-profile project, particularly one which allows you to get seen by different parts of the business.

The wonderful thing about the menopause and this time of life, if we approach it in a positive way, is that it gives us more confidence. We worry less about what people think, we are better able to be assertive, asking for what we want and standing up for what we believe in and we can begin to finally accept who we are. Who would want the angst of being 17 again?!

I believe that we should not deny the fact that we are reaching the menopausal years; don't hide it, but don't talk about it all the time either. If you act as if it is just a normal occurrence, so will everyone else.

Strategies

Here are some strategies that I have learned to help me cope at work with the symptoms of the menopause:

- When I have a hot flush and I think people may have noticed, I laugh and say in the lightest of tones, "Oh! I am having a hot moment!" and smile, then I carry on as if nothing has happened. I've also heard it called a 'tropical moment'. Besides, in the winter, some of my hot flushes have been a complete godsend, warming me up from head to toe – marvellous!

- My favourite tip is counting down from 360. Typically, a hot flush will last for about three minutes. When I'm in a situation where I cannot ignore the symptom, I just count. Surprisingly, I have never reached below 100. I start thinking about other things or doing something different.

- Remember just to focus on what you are doing and what you want to achieve, work out your priorities and then you know what to pay attention to; reserve some time in your diary to give yourself time to reflect. You might want to get your coach to help you to think it through and make an action plan

- Identify potential tricky situations. Decide beforehand how you will tackle them, work out how you are going to handle things and respond. Be flexible; if what you are doing isn't working, then do something else. Refine your strategy by trial and error.

- Find someone to talk to who is in a similar position to you, who will support you and help you to keep positive. This could be a colleague but perhaps even better to have someone outside of work who understands your situation. This needs to be someone you can trust and confide in.

Sometimes the symptoms of the menopause catch us unawares, and we might be lost for words or stuck for something to say. Here's an idea from a fellow participant on a training course. We were working as a pair on an activity and I was completely sidetracked by a really hot and, I felt, very noticeable flush. She told me that if that ever happened to her when she was in a one-to-one situation, she would say that she was really excited by being with the other person and that this showed in her physiology. She said she had been with a male colleague once when this had happened, she told him that she was very excited by the project they were working on, he looked a little taken aback and then she said to him, "Don't you feel like that too? It's marvellous, you should try it!" I thought that was the funniest thing. I've never actually used this as a technique, but I always have it available as an option.

The menopause is a time of big change for us, our bodies are not quite the same and some of us don't have the same drive and commitment to things that we previously found highly motivating. For working women, much of our time will be spent at work as we steer the way through our familiar landscape with a new perspective.

In the beginning, the onset of the menopause can bring shock, anxiety and fear, destabilising our entire life. Everything that we used to know about ourselves is evolving, and our way of dealing with life no longer seems to quite fit. Creating a new sense of self in amongst this upheaval takes a lot of guts and determination, but it definitely makes us stronger and we emerge on the other side, reborn with a new sense of power.

Chapter 13

Creating the Future

God, grant me the SERENITY to accept the things I cannot change, COURAGE to change the things I can; and WISDOM to know the difference

We have come to the last chapter and I have shared with you some ideas, tools, tips and techniques to enable you to think differently and to help you to handle the emotional side of the menopause. If you have not yet done so, perhaps now is the time to decide to get in the driving seat, take control and step into your power.

You have everything you need to take charge of your own life and destiny. Your determination and strength will see you through. Even on the days where you don't feel as strong as on others, you can remember that this is only a passing phase and you will soon be on the other side of it. We just get one life to live, so you might like to think about how you can make it a great one! You know that 'this is it'; as they say, it's not a rehearsal.

All you need to do is use the power of your own mind; as my mother used to say, "You can do it if you put your mind to it". You can decide to make this part of your life wonderful and enjoyable in spite of any physical symptoms you might have. However, it takes focus, persistence and determination; it might not happen if you just wish it, so you will need to take action, too.

Using your mind and being happy

Some women say when the menopause starts that they feel like they are going mad. That feeling of forgetting things, losing things and putting things in the wrong places is absolutely maddening. I'm trying to think of more examples, but I've forgotten them! I once wanted to make doubly sure that I had my glasses with me, so I put two pairs of glasses in my handbag. An hour later I set off, only to arrive at the venue to discover that I had no glasses. I then realised that I'd taken both pairs out of my bag for different reasons and hadn't replaced them. Bonkers, eh!

I really did think that I was showing signs of dementia; I would lose my words or I'd ask someone a question and, while I was waiting for the answer, I'd forget what my original question had been! It can be so embarrassing. But now I just shrug it off with a laugh. I have every faith that, once the hormones settle down, my brain will return to some sort of normality. Funnily enough, the more I stop trying to be perfect, and show vulnerability to others, the more I find people being open with me and they help me more, too. So my philosophy has become: Shrug it off with a laugh, it is not important, and in a little while it will not matter *at all*.

You can be happy every day, it's just a choice.

Robert Holden has a website devoted to happiness which I love to visit: www.happiness.co.uk. One of the inspirational messages I found on the site is 'Happiness is only one thought away'. I've heard a few women who, in spite of having lots of symptoms, say that they would far rather be alive and have the symptoms than the opposite. It all depends on your perspective and what you believe. As I've said already, be careful what you focus on, because that is what you will end up with.

I've noticed that today we have the religion of 'I want it, and I want it now' and hang the consequences. We want instant gratification without thinking about the longer term. Perhaps we should be firm with ourselves and think about the future but maybe occasionally, this self-indulgence might be totally appropriate at this time of life! This does not mean eating 25 doughnuts all at once just because you feel like it and forgetting about the waistline! I'm not saying that you should over-indulge yourself, but I am saying that you should make sure you make the most out of the life you have. Identify what happiness means to you and what will give you that: for example, the simple pleasures we spoke of in Chapter 11, the friendships and relationships, the hobbies or pastimes, the work that fulfils you, things that give you pleasure. You can be, and you deserve to be, happy.

Final thoughts

Here are what I consider to be the key messages that I would like to remind you of; if you want to handle the emotional side of the menopause, they will definitely help you to do a good job of it.

Give yourself time to think and adjust, be kind to yourself. It's a big deal, this change stuff, so make sure you give yourself some space and also cut yourself some slack. You don't have to strive for perfection; you are perfect as you are. You are the best 'you' that there is on the planet. No one can do 'you' as well as you can!

Make space too, by de-cluttering your mind, your home, and your work tasks. Forgive anyone whose behaviour requires it, not for their sake but for yours. Let go of negative emotions that you might have about others. Forgive them, forget and move on. They are doing their best in their own little world in the same way you are doing your best in yours.

Be selfish and take care of yourself – you need to make sure that you are in good shape to do all the things you want to do. You can make a big difference here with some small changes, like improving your diet, making sure you take exercise and making room for all those things that you meant to do but hadn't quite got round to.

Listen to your body: if it indicates thirst, drink water; if it signals tiredness, think twice before you remedy that with caffeine which masks how you feel. You already know that you are what you eat, and everyone needs a specific diet for themselves, so begin to notice which foods make you feel great and which drain the energy from you.

If you are finding it tough, maybe get some help from experts: nutritionists, homeopaths, massage therapists and acupuncturists can all offer different types of support. Work out which would give you the most benefit and give it a try.

Remember that it is a journey with stages, and despite the fact that many women have been there before you, this is your own rite of passage and no one will do it like you. On the one hand, you are on your own; on the other hand, there is a lot of support from people around you. Even a sympathetic smile from a woman you don't know, who notices the discomfort of a hot flush, can help you along your way. Take heart, you will come out the other end, still yourself and yet reborn in new way.

Notice your emotions and deal with them, recognising the effect they have, both on yourself and on others. Be honest about it and don't make excuses.

Lighten up, attitude is everything – look for the positive, look on the bright side, and be grateful for what you have.

It's time to get to the point where you run your own life, rather than it running you and, to do that, it helps if you are clear on the following:

What you want and where you are going

What you want in your life

What you want out of your life

What you want gone from your life

My life has completely turned around in the past few years since the beginning signs of the menopause. At one point, I can remember thinking, 'I've turned into a woman in comfortable shoes and I feel as if I'm going grey on the inside'. I was in a relationship yet I felt very alone. Although I was really scared of what would happen, I left my partner of 15 years, having decided that I would be happier on my own rather than in an unfulfilling relationship with someone who could not really give me what I needed. Looking back, I don't think either of us was happy, but we had fallen into a way of living together and hadn't really noticed that we had grown apart. I moved from the country back to the city – I never thought **that** would ever happen!

I reinvented myself: new hairstyle and new way of dressing. All of that gave me a new sense of self which was wonderful. Then, to my utter amazement, I met the love of my life the following Christmas. I had never dreamed that it was possible to find someone who was so perfect for me and vice versa. Eighteen months later, we were married and are planning on living happily ever after.

It wasn't easy and there were tough decisions to make, but I have come through it, I think a better person, and I am happier now than I have ever been.

So I leave you with this thought: Who knows what could happen when you relax and let your new self emerge? Don't let these symptoms get the better of you, take charge, look to the future and do what you want. Have what you wish for. Be everything you can be.

It might be a bumpy ride, but why not make it worth the effort. After all, you only get this one precious life; it's up to you what you make of it.

Optional Extra

The next chapter is a bonus one which is written for the man in your life, if you have one. I know that some people will not have a man around right now, but you never know ...

It is meant for a man who may not want to read the whole book but would like some insight and some helpful tips. (Perhaps you could leave it open at the appropriate page, or insert a bookmark.)

Bonus Chapter

For men

*"All changes, even the most longed for, have their
melancholy; for what we leave behind us is a
part of ourselves; we must die to one
life before we can enter another"*

Anatole France

This chapter is particularly for the man whose wife,
girlfriend, partner or significant other is approaching or
going through the menopause. Sometimes it is the people
around the woman involved who notice the pre-menopausal
or menopausal symptoms first.

Technically the menopause starts when periods have stopped
for a year; before that time, women who have the symptoms of
menopause are in the perimenopause.

*Stephen told me that he thinks his wife is going mad. She is
argumentative, angry, impatient and she rows and shouts,
which she never did before. He is at his wits' end and is
considering leaving because he can't stand it any longer; he
hates going home and spends more and more time in the
office. They have a teenage son who is going through puberty;
Stephen says his home life is a nightmare. It's possible that
she is perimenopausal, but he does not want to bring up the
topic in case it starts another row.*

So, first and foremost, here are the symptoms; it can include any of the following:

1. Aches and pains

2. Anxiety, feeing ill at ease, feelings of dread, apprehension, doom

3. Bone damage, Osteoporosis (often after several years)

4. Breast tenderness

5. Burning tongue, burning roof of mouth, bad taste in mouth

6. Changes in eating patterns

7. Changes in fingernails (density, softness, cracking, etc.)

8. Crashing fatigue and sudden tiredness

9. Depression

10. Difficulty concentrating, disorientation, mental confusion

11. Disrupted sleep patterns, trouble sleeping through the night (not always because of night sweats)

12. Disturbing memory lapses or loss

13. Dizziness, light-headedness, episodes of loss of balance

14. Dry eyes

15. Electric shock sensation under the skin and in the head

16. Exacerbation of existing conditions

17. Eyesight changes

18. Frequent urination

19. Gastrointestinal distress, indigestion, flatulence, gas pain, nausea, feeling bloated

20. Hair loss or thinning – head, pubic, or whole body; increase in facial hair

21. Headaches

22. Heavy periods, irregular periods

23. Hot flushes

24. Incontinence

25. Increase in allergies

26. Increased tension in muscles

27. Irritability

28. Lack of energy

29. Loss of libido

30. Mood swings, sudden emotional shifts

31. Night sweats then may feel cold, often associated with a clammy feeling

32. Skin irritation, itchy, dry, and/or crawly skin

33. Tingling in the extremities

34. Tinnitus: ringing in ears, bells, ringing, buzzing etc.

35. Urinary infections

36. Vaginal dryness

37. Vaginal infections

38. Weight gain or loss

Women can suffer some, all or none of these symptoms. About 15% of women have no symptoms, their periods stop and that's it. Every single woman is different and, just to make it more complicated, every day can be different, too. So if you were hoping for predictability and order, then this is probably not the time you will find it!

I have about 12 of these symptoms, not all at the same time. The most noticeable are the hot flushes and the night sweats which are undeniable symptoms of the menopause. Some of the others could be caused by something else. The most debilitating for me is the loss of concentration; sometimes I feel really fuzzy-headed and find it difficult to think clearly. It is so frustrating.

It took me a while to realise that the tiredness was down to the menopause; At times I am just too tired to do anything. I can wake up after a fairly good night's sleep feeling as if I need another four hours. Then I feel guilty because I don't want to do anything and I've got a great long list of 'shoulds' to do. This is compounded when I do very little on some days and feel bad because I have wasted so much time.

The flip side of that is if I do too much I get even more tired, everything seems to be very difficult and hard to do, then I make mistakes and get ratty and grumpy because it stresses me out. Hmmm … a no-win situation!

I wish I had appreciated all that spare time I had in my teens, when I would wish away great swathes of time, looking forward to a party or the weekend or a holiday. Now every moment seems too precious to waste, and that creates pressure too.

I asked some male friends a few questions about their experience of the menopause; these are the questions:

1. What do you think about how the menopause affects women?

2. What has been your experience of the menopause?

3. Has it ever been a problem for someone close to you? And were you able to help?

4. Can you offer any helpful suggestions for other men who may be dealing with a menopausal woman?

5. Any other thoughts you think might be useful?

This is what my friend Alex wrote:

1. What do you think about how the menopause affects women?

I think there are two aspects, from personal experience: one is the physical and one is the mental.

Physically, my wife has experienced a lot of the unpleasant symptoms, such as hot flushes, aches and pains; this does get her down and makes her irritable with the family. She won't take HRT because of the cancer risk. I try to sympathise with her complaints but it can be tough as this has been going on for ages (does it ever end?)

Mentally there are days when I wonder who I am living with. It is just like friend to fiend, as she goes from being a kind, thoughtful, loving person who becomes emotional, shouts a lot, hectors me and the children, and nags incessantly until I have to speak to her quietly and tell her I am not prepared to accept such abuse any more, which seems to at least quieten her down. When it first started, I used to shout back (and if under stress, occasionally still do). Once I realised the cause, I was able to at least adjust my response but it is hard for the children and they have started to shout back.

It hasn't been helped by my daughter starting her periods last year. It's like being between two banshees if the cycles coincide!

At times, it feels like a war zone and I just want to find a quiet place but won't leave the children to suffer unless I am away.

To be honest, at one point I thought she was mentally ill and suggested she might see someone, but then realised it wasn't happening all the time.

2. What has been your experience of the menopause?

As above ... plus my mother went through it and I know my father suffered similarly. With her, however, it was exacerbated by drinking a bit too much and I can recall lying in bed and just wishing the shouting would end.

3. And were you able to help?

To help, I am beginning to understand that I can:

Take the kids away for a couple of hours and give her and us some space (but then she'll often complain that I am stopping them from doing homework!)

Try and listen, which can sometimes be difficult when working from home or walking in after a hard day at work.

4. Can you offer any helpful suggestions for other men who may be dealing with a menopausal woman?

Listen. Don't escalate the arguments; let her articulate all her frustration and anger. I guess there must be some anguish at knowing you won't have any more kids and you are getting older.

Get her to explain what it is all about, maybe get us to look it up and understand it more.

Let us know early so we know what the hell is happening.

Try and get some humour involved. One tactic I try when we start getting irritable is to smile after I have said something in an argument; we both end up smiling and things calm down.

Remember that under this dragon skin is the woman you love!

5. Any other thoughts you think might be useful?

Hmm. I wonder if sometimes it isn't used as a bit of an excuse for bad behaviour (don't shoot me). I wonder if you can get over to women the anguish it is causing men, too. Here is someone they have loved for years and suddenly it is like sharing the house with a new person and not one you would have married (I wonder if it is why some men run off with younger women?) Don't try and hide it through embarrassment, tell the man what is happening quickly, as mentioned.

Alex is by no means the only person to have had a similar experience with his wife. So take heart, you are not alone and there is an end to it, though things might be different when you come out the other side.

The male 'midlife crisis'

You might like to consider that men go through their own 'mid-life crisis'. Whilst it doesn't have to be a crisis, this time of life brings up issues for men as well as women. The growing paunch, thinning hair, eyesight not as great as it was and reducing levels of testosterone affect men in a somewhat similar way to women. And there's a name for it too: Andropause. Here are some of the symptoms:

- Problems with erections

- Low sex drive

- Moods, including depression and irritability

- Feeling tired

- Loss of muscle size and strength

- Osteoporosis (bone thinning)

- Increased body fat

- Difficulty with concentration and memory loss

- Sleep difficulties

The onset of the andropause is much less noticeable than the menopause. The symptoms sneak up on men, whereas some women, including me, say the change of life hit them like a train.

It might be easy to put the reason for any emotional problems squarely at the door of the menopause, but it is possible that both people may be experiencing changes. I wonder whether, unwittingly, we blame the emotional difficulties on the menopause when there might be other factors to take into account as well.

This time of life brings changes to both parties, and it's worth remembering that the man might also need some time and space to think more fully about this and consider what is important in his life and where he is going. There are many activities described in the book that you can do to help you to look anew at your situation.

Here is how Robert described how this time of life has affected him:

Loss of some sleep. Awareness that someone is going through change which, to an extent, signals one's own journey through life. A recognition that things are changing for oneself. For me, a change in priorities. Counting the years to the end rather than from the beginning. Less ambitious. Wanting to do things away from work. In many ways wanting to control one's own life and to focus on things that really matter and that you can do before the end, rather than trying to keep up with one's siblings or friends etc. In other words, the effects are more spiritual than physical; although one needs to understand that one's own libido is changing.

Handling your own emotions

There are a number of techniques in the book to help you to handle your emotions. You'll find a list of them on page 231.

The first thing is to recognise your emotions and how they affect how you behave.

For example, Michael comes home from work, he is tired and feeling annoyed because he has been let down again by the project manager. Kathy, his wife, has had numerous hot flushes that day and is feeling tense and edgy; she had palpitations earlier in the day and is worried that it might be something serious. As she begins to talk to Michael about all this, he is in no mood to listen, he just wants some peace and quiet to read the paper and watch the news. She gets frustrated and annoyed with him, thinking that he is insular, selfish and uncaring. She starts banging about in the kitchen, slamming doors and making lots of noise ... the row is ready to begin ... escalation ... shouting ... sulking ... getting things on an even keel again ... both disturbed by the argument, feeling shaky and stressed.

This argument did not help either of the people in the situation and yet neither was able to realise this and stop the fight. Had they been able to keep calm, manage their emotions and have a conversation about it, things would have been easier all round.

We all know how destructive this negative behaviour is, and we have probably all said things we regret in the heat of the moment, words that cannot be taken back. Sometimes people say things that wound in the moment, but that also linger and hurt for months and years afterwards. Right now, if you stop to think about it for a short time, you can probably recall something nasty said to you years ago in anger that you still remember and that still hurts.

Sometimes we get into these situations or arguments because we want to win, or because we don't want *them* to win, or because we've got to have the last word or because we've got to be right. These reasons hijack our ability to see the bigger picture, and cause us to lose sight of who the other person is. We forget that actually we are fighting with someone we love, over something that might be trivial, even though at the time it seems vitally important. Worst of all, we lose respect for the other person and stop treating them like a human being with feelings; they become 'the enemy'.

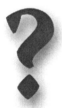

What emotions cause you to lose control?

In what situations do you let your emotions get the better of you?

Once you recognise your trigger points, you can stop and think rationally about what is going on and how you want to handle it, rather than letting the emotion take over (the freeze-frame technique in Chapter 3 is brilliant for this, and is definitely worth practising).

Here are 4 top tips:

1 Pay attention to your thoughts and behaviours and notice when your emotions are running the show.

2. Keep control of your emotions.

3. Let go of the need to win or have the last word. Look for a win-win for both of you.

4. The old favourite: Count to 10 slowly to give yourself time to think.

Creating a new life together

Whether you like it or not, her change signals a change for you, too. You might prefer to hang on to the status quo and seek refuge in your habitual ways of doing things but, because she is evolving, you cannot stay the same. If the way she feels causes a change in her behaviour, then it is likely that it will cause a change in your behaviour as well. This, in turn, will have an impact on the partnership and the life you have together.

We can look at the menopause from the perspective of 'Systems thinking'. This is a theory or a methodology that originated in cybernetics which can also be used for problem-solving. It involves looking at a situation considering the whole picture, as opposed the seeing a small part in isolation. Often we focus on small details and we don't notice the entire situation or consider who or what else might be affected.

If you change one element of a 'system' it has a knock-on effect on everything else in that 'system'. It also affects the way the 'system' works as a whole.

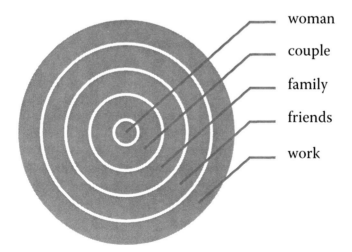

woman

couple

family

friends

work

Here is how this relates to the menopause. Let's say we are talking about one single menopausal symptom, which is part of a set of symptoms. Each of these symptoms affects the whole of her system (i.e. her body and mind) which, in turn, is part of a greater system (her family). From a systems perspective, she is one element in a bigger system – that of a couple, or a family for example. (There are also wider systems around those: the community and the workplace are also systems that she functions within.)

We can take the example of my night sweats which are just a symptom for me. Here is how they affect the system that I am in: I get overheated at night and need a change of pyjamas, therefore I have to do more laundry and I must find time for that so it impacts on any time schedule that I might have for my day. My sleep gets disrupted, so I lose sleep, then I am more tired in the morning, I get irritated more easily which affects everyone around me, plus I am stressed because I've got extra washing to do. I feel overloaded and also I don't concentrate as well when I'm tired, so my work suffers, too. All this makes me even more stressed, then I wind myself up about whether I'll be able to sleep or not ... meanwhile, the people around me experience me as ineffective, neurotic, tired and grumpy!

Therefore, if a woman's symptoms are causing changes in her, then that will have a knock-on effect and will change the relationships with the people around her.

Some examples of this systems thinking are as follows:

- Two people live happily together, they have a baby and the whole way their life works has to change to accommodate the child. They cannot stay the same and do the same things and raise a child effectively.

- The child grows up and leaves home to go to university, comes back during the holidays and then comes back home again to live. At each stage, the system (and by that

I mean all the people in the scenario) changes in response to the differing circumstances.

- An even simpler example: let's say someone gives you a big, heavy-duty stew pot as a present. You might find that your whole kitchen cupboard system has to be reorganised to accommodate it!

Here is an activity to enable you to map out your own 'system'. (You can do this individually, or you could do it as a couple).

Activity: Mapping myself and my system

Time: 15 minutes

Kit: Paper and pen

Write up a list of the people and areas that make up your 'system' - I would suggest no more than eight to start with.

Examples might include: Home, Health and Fitness, Marriage/Relationship, Friends, Family, Spirituality, Work, Personal Development, Finances, Leisure Time, Time for Me, Community.

Take a sheet of paper and draw a circle about four inches in diameter in the middle of it. Divide the circle into 'slices' according to how many important areas of life you have. Label each slice. Give each area a score out of 10, (one being low, 10 being high) as to how satisfied you are with that area of your life. Colour in the appropriate size of slice.

Here's an example of how it might look:

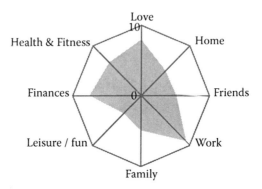

You can then think about the system of your life, looking at each area and how it impacts the others.

For the example above, you might say that the person is spending a lot of time on work and finances and seems to be missing out on friends and leisure and fun.

Using this structured approach, you can begin to think about which areas are working well and identify those where you would like to make some changes.

Five ways to support her

1. Don't blame, judge or compare – just accept

2. Communicate

3. Listen

4. Help

5. Compliment

Don't blame, judge or compare

I can't imagine that anyone would wish to be at this time of life, with all the changes, discomfort and emotions that it brings. It might be tempting to look for someone to blame, to make it someone's fault or to lay the responsibility somewhere, but it is irrelevant and unhelpful. She did not ask for it and most likely, would prefer it if it were not happening. Be careful not to judge her harshly and also avoid comparison with either her 'old self' or with other women around her. Every woman will feel, look and act differently. Just take her as she is and appreciate her and love her. Let her know you are on her side, whatever happens. This will do a lot to ease any tension she might feel about how you feel about her.

Communication

It is critical that you talk to each other while you are going through this; that you share how you feel and what you think, without blaming or judging each other. This is not the time to score points or make sure you are right.

Talk about the symptoms and learn more about it – not to show off your great knowledge to her, but to help you to understand what it is all about. It's bewildering to be having all these unfamiliar physical symptoms. Some of them are quite frightening. For example: before I realised that palpitations were a symptom, there was one particular afternoon where I was absolutely convinced I was about to die.

Listen

In general, men do not like to see their woman unhappy, and they want to find a solution to the problem quickly, to fix it and make it go away. From the female perspective, this approach can make her feel as if he is not interested in what is going on for her, and that he just wants to make it go away because it is tiresome and he is fed up with it. Like any advice we might get from someone, it has to fit the person, and they need to be ready to hear it. So, you have to be careful of trying to fix things because it suggests lack of patience and interest and, even though the original intention was to make the woman feel better and happier, often it doesn't have the desired effect.

A more effective approach is to work together to find how to deal with it, to help her to come up with the solutions. And by the way, I don't mean that *you* have worked out the answer yourself and you just get her to discover the solution you wanted her to come up with. What you need to do is to be really open and listen; as Alex said, to really listen to her and hear what she is saying and how she is feeling and get a sense of this new perspective she is dealing with. It's not only the physical symptoms that are at play here, but also the emotional side.

She has to come to terms with a whole new way of being, a new identity, a new self, a new body. A feeling of lack of femininity, looks changing, no more children, the stark realisation that it is nearer the end of life than the beginning. Whereas before there was everything to look forward to, now there is a worry that there is so little left.

It's a steep learning-curve and, for most women, one that they would rather not be on, thank you very much.

Listen to her to help her discover what this new self is like and, of course, for you to discover it, too.

This may be a sweeping generalisation but, in my opinion, men have an ability to listen in a way that is rather particular to that sex. It's almost as if they have a little tape-recorder in their ear which allows them to record what has been said without actually listening properly. Then, when challenged by wife/girlfriend/partner/significant other who says in a very loud voice, or even a shout, "You're not listening to me!", the man is able to repeat the last few sentences of what was said, verbatim but without actually having really listened, taken in or processed any of the information in their own brain.

It is a VERY IRRITATING habit or ability! If I can also add, it does not constitute good listening etiquette and if you would like some advice: **do not do it!**

Tips

Do not try to listen and multi-task at the same time! Don't be half-reading the paper or watching football out of the corner of your eye!

Give her time to think it through – you might not want to hear it all, but you have no idea how helpful it is for her if you just listen.

Be curious about how her thought patterns are working.

Don't try to look for solutions while you are listening – it is not really up to you to find the solution, even though you would like to. It is for her to find out for herself.

Consider this: she is like a chrysalis, so be gentle.

Be patient, it is not all going to be over in one conversation.

Remember this is something that affects both of you, not just her.

Ask questions

You might need to be brave and ask things that you are not sure you want to know the answer to! But it helps if you find out how she is feeling; also the questions you ask her will help her to think about it.

Learn to be comfortable with silence while she thinks about what you have asked. It might be tempting to jump in and provide the answers for her, but just give her time to think.

Take care with how you phrase the questions. For example, asking, "Are you feeling awful again today?" is likely to result in her thinking about the negatives of the situation which, by the way, she might not have been thinking about before you asked! Try to ask questions in such a way that it could lead her to thinking in a more positive way.

If, for example, she says that she is very tired, you could ask, "What kind of tired?" Then, if appropriate after the answer, you might ask, "What do you want to do about that?" Or you could just say gently, "Tell me about it". (Be really careful with your tone of voice when you ask these questions – the idea is to sound caring and interested).

Help

This is so obvious but perhaps worth mentioning anyway. As the 'system' of your life together is changing, then your routines and habits may change too. Take another look at how you share the chores and make sure they are shared out equitably. Sometimes just a small gesture of help makes all the difference. Take a new look at how you can help each other.

Compliments

Remember to tell her when she looks lovely – don't just think it, say it. It is so important for us to know we are still attractive, in spite of our maturing faces and bodies. You can improve her confidence and her mood with an honest, positive comment. Do not underestimate how valuable this is.

Stephen thinks Christine (49) is very attractive, she gets lots of admiring glances when she is out, he assumes that she knows that she looks great and rarely bothers to tell her. When she asks him how she looks, for example when they are dressed up and ready to go out, he says, "You look fine". She does not see herself as attractive and doesn't notice the glances of others; her self-confidence is diminishing as her looks begin to fade. She says she is beginning to feel like a nobody. She starts to let herself go because who cares anyway?

Peter thinks Linda (52) is very attractive, he is very proud of her and frequently tells her when he likes how she looks or how she is dressed. He always seems to be on the look-out for things about her that he loves. He notices her clothes, hair and make-up. Because of this, she makes an effort to look good, which he then compliments. She knows that she is changing physically but she copes with it well because of the positive attention she gets from Peter.

Stephen and Christine have been together for 16 years, Peter and Linda for only three years. Perhaps time and familiarity have made Stephen and Christine pay less attention to each other as individuals with feelings, both of them probably need reassurance from time to time.

You might like to stop and think for a few minutes about:

How much attention and positive feedback do you give?

How much you would like to receive?

How could you have a conversation to talk about this?

And in closing

What will you do differently as a result of reading this?

*"The happiness of life is made up of minute fractions –
the little, soon forgotten charities of a kiss or a smile,
a kind look or heartfelt compliment"*

Samuel Taylor Coleridge

Techniques and Websites

Freeze frame   p. 43

Three chairs   p. 53

Making a mind map   p. 68

Visualisation   p. 100

Generative writing   p. 109

The GROW model   p. 188

http://www.happiness.co.uk

http://www.brainsync.com

http://www.pzizz.com

http://www.heartmath.org

http://www.thinkbuzan.com

http://www.menopausesupport.org.uk

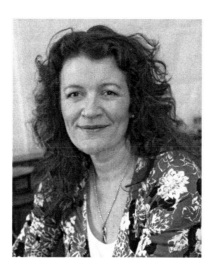

Barbara Frodsham has devoted most of her professional life to helping people achieve their potential. In the past 20 years she has trained and coached hundreds of individuals to enable them to handle their challenges and problems more effectively, including a 100% success rate with clients who are looking for a promotion at work. "Much of the key to unlocking these problems involves a shift in mental attitude along with building confidence and self-esteem" she says. Many of her clients find her motivational and inspirational.

Barbara is Managing Director of Loxwood Interactive Ltd., working with individuals and organisations to make the most of their talent, knowledge and experience.

She is a qualified executive coach, with an Advanced Diploma in Professional Coaching and Mentoring, a Master Practitioner and Trainer of Neuro-Linguistic Programming (NLP), a qualified NLP coach, Master Practitioner of Hypnotherapy, trained in Thought Field Therapy, Archetypal Branding, Symbolic Modeling and numerous psychological models.

Member of the British Psychological Society and the International Coach Federation.

www.loxwood.co.uk
www.momentouscoaching.com

Lightning Source UK Ltd.
Milton Keynes UK
31 August 2010

159216UK00001B/2/P